*More praise for*
# A PIECE OF MY MIND

"A collection of short, often dramatic pieces that offer the reader a rare opportunity to share the secret internal world of the physician . . . A book that can be read and enjoyed by physicians and nonphysicians alike."

*Facets*

"Readers wishing to expand their moral imaginations—physicians, patients, medical scholars; or anyone—will find here enchanting interlocutors."

*American Journal of Psychiatry*

# A PIECE
# OF MY MIND

## A Collection of Essays from
## *The Journal of the*
## *American Medical Association*

Edited by
Dr. Bruce B. Dan
and Roxanne K. Young
With and introduction and commentary by
Dr. Bruce B. Dan
and a foreword by
Dr. Art Ulene

BALLANTINE BOOKS • NEW YORK

# CONTENTS

# CONTENTS

# ACKNOWLEDGMENTS

Thanks to the following persons, without whose efforts this collection could not have come to fruition:

Helga Wutz, editorial assistant, *JAMA*, who not only ensures that "A Piece of My Mind" appears each week but who also deftly processes 700 manuscript rejections each year; Lawrence D. Grouse, M.D., Ph.D., who kept the column going during its formative years; Toinette Lippe, our editor, who pulled it all together; and Mori Bombyx, whose creativity provided the inspiration for the book.

# FOREWORD

When the husband of a seriously ill patient turns to you for reassurance, how do you hide the fact that you are just as frightened as he is about the way his wife's disease is progressing? How do you hold out hope without being dishonest?

When a child is dying of an incurable disorder, how do you cope with your inability to cure him? When his mother comes to you for comfort and support, how do you conceal your own grief and tears?

When you make an error and a patient suffers for it, how do you keep self-doubts from interfering with your care of other patients afterward? How do you prevent self-recriminations from taking the joy out of your work?

When a patient sues you over a bad result—in spite of the fact that there were no errors in his care—how do you keep your rage from spoiling relationships with other patients? How do you stop yourself from ordering unnecessary tests in self-defense?

These are the questions that practicing physicians must answer for themselves every day. These questions reflect a side of medicine that few people except physicians are aware of, and few want to hear about. It is discomfiting for people who grew up with Marcus Welby to discover that real doctors have doubts and fears, and that they don't know all the answers.

But that's the way real doctors are, and that's why I found myself so powerfully drawn to "A Piece of My Mind." These essays describe with sometimes chilling honesty what real doctors think and feel; they reflect what I have been experiencing myself for more than 25 years. *A Piece of My Mind* contains a piece of every physician; it contains a piece of me.

These essays were written to be read by doctors. In sharing them more widely now, there is a slight risk that others will learn how much like them we physicians are. It's a risk worth taking. The more honest physicians can be with their patients, the more effective we can be as healers, and the more comfortable we can be as humans.

Art Ulene, M.D.

# INTRODUCTION

The "A Piece of My Mind" column was inaugurated in May 1980 in *The Journal of the American Medical Association* *(JAMA)* by the late Sam Vaisrub, M.D., in an editorial entitled "For the Peace of Your Mind." Dr. Vaisrub's announcement of this departure from the usual scientific and technical articles appearing in the weekly medical journal was accompanied by the first essay published ("Tuna on Rye, 1984"), under Dr. Vaisrub's pen name, Sam Vee.

Since then the weekly column has been the most popular section in what is now the world's most widely circulated medical journal. Under the direction of *JAMA*'s Associate Editor, Roxanne K. Young, the column has succeeded admirably in its original goal—to let doctors share with each other their most moving experiences, the human side of medicine.

More than 425 essays and poems have been published to date, but almost 4500 manuscripts, including poetry and even drawings, have been submitted in hope of publication. Currently *JAMA* receives almost 800 unsolicited submissions a year, and chooses only 50 for publication. We believe the overwhelming popularity of the column stems from the fact that doctors are given the opportunity to divulge some of their most deeply held feelings, perhaps for the first time in their lives. It is also of no small consequence to each author that *JAMA* has a worldwide circulation of more than 650,000. *The Journal* appears in seven foreign languages and in more than 140 other countries. "A Piece of My Mind" essays have appeared in virtually all of the non-English editions at one time or another.

In the last several years the lay public has discovered "A

Piece of My Mind'' too. Essays have been reprinted in dozens of newspapers, magazines, newsletters, the *Reader's Digest*, and even other medical journals.

It should be no surprise that *JAMA* receives a continuous stream of letters commenting on the column, but they are not just from physicians. Many come from family members who have seen *The Journal* in a physician's home and read the column, or from patients who have picked up a copy in their doctor's office. But in the last several years *JAMA* has been getting more and more letters asking for a collection of the essays to be published in a book. Clearly it was time to gather together the very best of ''A Piece of My Mind'' and let everyone share in what shouldn't be a secret—that doctors feel deeply about their profession and about the people who have entrusted their health and their lives to them.

Because the articles were originally essays written for other physicians, they often contain words of technical meaning, medical jargon, and esoteric abbreviations. There is a glossary of terms at the back of the book which I hope will make most of the potentially confusing terms clear.

While the essays themselves stand on their own, I have included a few personal comments throughout the book. I have also included letters and other comments published in *JAMA* in response to some of the more provocative essays of ''A Piece of My Mind.''

Here, then, are 80 personal glimpses of medicine from the people who live in that world every day. This is as real as it gets.

Bruce B. Dan, M.D.
Chicago, 1988

# BABY BLUES

## Daniel J. Waters, D.O.

More than anything, it's the eyes that haunt you. All at once full of wonder, bewildered, yet somehow accusing. You can see almost anything you want in them if you look long enough. Trust perhaps? Or is it resignation? A glimmer of understanding that seems to vanish in an instant.

It's always the eyes you remember.

They lie in a sea of high-powered technology, some rocking gently on the water mattresses meant to simulate the womb from which they were thrust too fast, too soon, unprepared, and ill equipped. Small clenched fists not grasping rattles or brightly colored toys, but arterial lines and plastic tubing. Silent cries from babies whose first pacifier is an endotracheal tube.

This is the world of an infant intensive care unit, a fluorescent, timeless place where children cry without sound and lullabies are barely audible above the gentle whoosh of the ventilators and the rhythmic beeping of the cardiac monitors.

We make our daily rounds, glibly discussing the T-E fistula in three or the possible NEC in six, gently probing tiny abdomens, listening to the harsh crackles of immature lungs straining to expand, checking the rapid patter of hearts no larger than a silver dollar. We adjust infusion rates, calculate fluid balance, and estimate maintenance requirements for bodies whose entire blood volume would fit in a teacup.

Across the room, two parents watch silently as their child gives a sleepy yawn, oblivious to the array of gauges and alarms that tell of the precarious balance in which this new life hangs. A furry stuffed toy nuzzles gently below a subclavian catheter line. An oversized baseball cap sits unabashedly atop a recent craniotomy.

As I peer up from a clipboard chock full of "the numbers" on each of my newborn charges, I find a pair of crystal blue eyes peering intently into my own. For a moment, I feel compelled to apologize, to justify, to explain why all this is necessary. I place my finger in the tiny palm to be reassured by the grasp reflex, which somehow doesn't seem quite so primitive right now. The eyes close in seeming silent understanding.

From isolette to isolette, each time it's the same. Always the eyes.

Placing my stethoscope on the chest of a sleeping 28-weeker, I'm met with another pair of questioning eyes.

"Where am I?" they seem to ask.

ICU, little one. A place that someday, when you're strong and healthy, you'll never remember.

ICU, little one. Can you really see me?

# AN APPLE FOR THE DOCTOR

## Lorenzo G. Guzman, M.D.

It had been a particularly vexing and difficult day. It was my birthday, and I was on the orthopedic surgery rotation of my general surgery residency. A few months before, the nursing personnel and the operating room supervisor had presented the chief resident on his birthday with a large ice cream cake and several useful gifts. I had taken careful notes and, when the time came, adeptly dropped a few casual remarks about my forthcoming birthday, making sure the exact date was properly fixed in the right people's minds.

The day came and there was no cake, no gifts, not even a remembrance or greeting card from anyone. I had had to assist in the operating room, first with a laborious hemipelvectomy, then with the repair of a torn shoulder rotator cuff, which had started long after the usual hour for planned surgical procedures. I misplaced the key to my operating room locker, and it had taken 45 minutes to retrieve same.

I had barely had time to cool off and organize myself to make evening rounds when the unit nurse burst into the office and bellowed, "Your patient in bed 1, ward C, refused his evening meal and smashed the dishes on the floor—there are spaghetti and coffee all over the place. That's more than I can take today!" Immediately I knew who she was talking about.

He was a 6-ft 9-in giant, 18 years old, who played center for the basketball team of his high school. A couple of months before, he had fractured his left upper arm in a rather trivial accident on the Bayonne—Staten Island Ferry. An x-ray film showed a tumor of the head of the humerus, biopsy of which revealed a primary osteosarcoma. A chest film showed multiple, bilateral seedings of the tumor, even in the chest wall. We had started chemotherapy, and, while the therapeutic response had been minimal, the side effects of the drugs had taken their allowable toll. He was anemic, weak, bald, and given to outbursts of ill temper. Somehow he had become attached to me, and I made it a point to chat with him every night after rounds. He didn't seem to understand his predicament and at times acted like a spoiled child.

All of the grievances and misfortunes of a sad day seemed to climax, and I shot out of my office, followed by the nurse and the junior residents and interns.

"Listen, you punk," I shouted angrily even before I reached his bed. "Let this be the last time you pull a stunt like this. If you do this again I'll have your can out of this place so fast you won't even know what hit you! Now you help the orderly clean up this mess and report to my office as soon as you finish." The tirade caught him by surprise, and after I thought I had duly impressed the nurse, the ward, and the other physicians, I avoided a confrontation by getting back to my office as quickly as I could.

I told the residents and interns that I was in no shape or mood to make rounds and that I would review the charts of the new admissions only. I had barely settled into the chair to proceed with my intended purpose when I heard a soft knock on the door. I grunted, and in walked the giant with a big, glossy, red apple in his hand.

"I found out today was your birthday," he said, as he appeared to measure his every word for fear of an interruption. I looked at him, seeing what the chemotherapy had done to him, and for a moment had thoughts about survivors of a concentration camp. I was emotionally disarmed and hated myself for having lost control a little earlier. "I saved this nice apple from my lunch, and I thought I'd give it to you as a birthday present. It really isn't much, but it's a very nice apple, and it's everything I got." I felt cheap, small, and undeserving. The petty grievances I had held against the world for not remembering my birthday seemed foolish, ridiculous, and stupid.

"Sit down, you big lug," I said. "This apple is the most beautiful present one could ever hope to receive. I simply love it."

My patient died three weeks later, and I went to his funeral in New Jersey. On the way back I thought about my birthday present, and how from that moment on it was to be a beacon in my search for the real values in patients and in human beings.

# MOLLY

## Peter D. Rogers, M.D., MPH

Molly Casey was blond and small and had eight freckles on her nose. She had brilliant green eyes and the middle of her upper lip was pinched just a little and turned up as if she were always preparing to kiss someone. Molly had been my patient since she was 12.

Molly had a way of getting things she wanted. She called them her "routines." Her "Camille routine" was used when she was sick. It was a series of emotive posturings that made it seem as if her death was imminent. I saw her use it convincingly once in my office in front of her mother. I never saw what she called her "Mary Poppins routine" or, after she read *Catcher in the Rye*, her "Holden Caulfield routine."

During one of Molly's office visits when she was 15, her mother complained that she couldn't get Molly "out of blue jeans and T shirts. That's all she'll wear. We make good money."

Molly responded to parental pressure with passive resistance—her "Mahatma Gandhi routine."

As Molly got older, it was apparent she was going to stay a small person. At 17, she was 5 ft 1 in and 95 lb, slightly smaller than her mother. Her brother, at age 18, was over 6 ft tall.

"When you're 5 ft 1, no one takes you seriously," she said to me when she was 16. "People tell me I'm cute. I

5

don't want to be cute. I want to be beautiful. When I get mad, they want to pat me on the head. I'm everybody's kid sister. My brother calls me 'Shortness.' I'm going to punch him the next time he calls me that. I really will."

"You know," she said as she was about to leave my office, "you're one of the few people who listen to me. I mean you *really* listen. I like that."

As young adulthood approached, Molly began to observe the rites of passage of that awkward time. She used a few drugs, smoked marijuana, drank.

A few days after her 17th birthday Molly asked me for a prescription for birth control pills.

"I didn't know you were sexually active, Molly."

"I'm not," she said angrily. "But I'm scouting around. Virginity is about as much fun as starvation."

Three months before her graduation from high school, Molly charged into my office.

"I'm leaving home," she proclaimed. "I'm getting out of here. I'm not getting along with my parents or my brother. Everybody has an idea of what I should be. They tell me what to say, how to act, what school to go to. They don't like my friends.

"I'm leaving. I'm going to California. They let you be a person out there. I never want to see or talk to my parents again. Never."

I tried to talk her out of going, but she had her mind made up.

"I have my plane ticket for LA. I'm leaving tonight."

As she started to leave my office, I called out to her.

"Molly, promise you'll call me at least once a month while you're gone. Let me keep your parents informed. Please."

She hesitated for a moment, nodded her head, and left.

Molly kept her promise for the next four months. The third time she called, her mood was euphoric. She was high on something. The fourth and last time she called, Molly was slurring her words and said something about "living with a guy." I pleaded with her to come home and told her that her parents desperately missed her. She laughed and hung up on me.

Six months passed and no one heard from her. It was an early December evening and we were getting our first snowfall. I was alone in my office preparing to go home. I heard someone come in the front door of the waiting room.

I walked out and saw a woman standing against the wall. She had no coat, wore a stained blue dress, and had shoes with inordinately high heels. Her long blond hair was matted. It was Molly. Her face was thin and drawn and she had a pained expression.

"I'm sick," she said in a weak voice. "Please help me."

I called her parents and took Molly to the emergency room.

She *was* sick.

I admitted her to the hospital with the diagnoses of gonorrhea with pelvic inflammatory disease and secondary syphilis.

I came into her room after her family had gone. She was sitting up in bed holding onto whatever defiance she still had.

I sat in a chair by her bed and we stared at each other. She looked so small and vulnerable.

"We're glad you're back, Molly. A lot of people around here love you."

"After what I've done?" she snapped. "I doubt it."

"You don't stop loving someone because they make a mistake."

"You know what my brother called me," she said, trying to sound angry. "He called me . . ." Her hand went to her eyes . . . her chest started heaving as she cried. "He called me 'Shortness.' I've . . . missed him . . . so much. My mom brought me some . . . of my old jeans . . . and T shirts. . . . I've missed my folks."

I took her hand.

"Please don't leave us again, Molly."

"Never . . . never . . . I promise." She wiped the tears from her cheeks with the back of her hand and I noticed her eight freckles. "I guess this is my 'Molly Casey routine.' "

I gave her hand a gentle squeeze, said good-night, and walked toward the door.

"Thanks for always being there when I needed you," she called to me. "And thanks . . . for now."

Molly never realized that I needed her more than she needed me. The world is full of doctors. There are precious few Molly Caseys.

# 'HI, LUCILLE, THIS IS DR. GOLD!'

## Lucille G. Natkins

I'm going in for a dilatation and curettage (D&C) next week. But even as I worry about carcinomas and five-year survival rates, an incident from my last D&C keeps popping into my mind.

That operation occurred after I hadn't seen a gynecologist in years. On my internist's recommendation I saw a physician whom I'll call Dr. James Gold, diplomate, American Board of Obstetrics and Gynecology; fellow, American College of Surgeons; and associate attending physician at a large teaching hospital. It turned out that he was a contemporary, that he lived in my neighborhood, and that his children and mine were classmates. He'd gone to medical school with one of my friends and interned with another. No one would have worried about inviting us to the same dinner party.

One visit and several phone calls later—all conducted on a cordial "Dr. Gold" and "Mrs. Natkins" basis—surgery was scheduled and soon afterward I was wheeled into the operating room. As my vision blurred and my legs numbed, a voice cut through the anesthetic haze. "Hi, Lucille, this is Dr. Gold!" Stupor turned to rage. "You expletive, that's not the way it goes! It goes 'Hi, Lucille, this is Jim' or 'Hi, Mrs. Natkins, this is Dr. Gold.'"

All soundless. I was out of it, zonked. The next thing I remember was a female voice saying "Wake up, Lucille, the operation's over. Wake up, Lucille." Damn, I thought, not again.

The biopsy findings were negative. I was free to stop worrying about gynecological malignancies, but "Hi, Lucille" wouldn't leave me. There are more dignified positions in life than lying naked and horizontal, legs spread-eagled, while half a dozen strangers shove their fists into what was once (wisely) called "one's private parts." But that indignity was unavoidable. What, though, was the purpose of "Hi, Lucille, this is Dr. Gold" from someone who would have been Jim had we met socially, or "Wake up, Lucille" from someone who was ensuring my waking by slapping my face? What purpose other than to underscore my lack of dignity and helplessness?

"Hi, Lucille" was still rankling months later when my 80-year-old mother-in-law was hospitalized. Overwhelmed by crippling arthritis and a host of other problems, she asked the nurse, whose name pin read "T. Bass," to "please get my slippers from the bedroom." "Whatever are you talking about, Bertha," snapped T. Bass, who was, perhaps, all of 30 years old. "You're in the hospital, not your house." My mother-in-law stiffened and blanched. Reality therapy with a bludgeon.

I became a first-name freak, asking friends and colleagues who addressed them by first name without expecting reciprocity and, conversely, whom they addressed by first name while expecting to be called Mr. Price or Dr. Wand. No surprises in this survey. Inferiors are called by first name: children, menial workers, the elderly, and women.

I wrote to the hospital where my mother-in-law had been a patient, noting that the hospital system that was reducing an 80-year-old woman to a child was robbing her of the will and determination she needed to ensure her recovery. The administrator replied that he could not understand my charges of abuse. I wrote to a widely syndicated medical columnist, asking why his replies to women began "Dear Amy" and to men "Dear Mr. Hall." No answer. "To the editor," I wrote a local paper. "It is demeaning to identify the county supervisor as 'Meg' while referring to males by surname or position." "To the editor," wrote the county supervisor. "It is endearing, and by no means demeaning, to be called 'Meg.' I enjoy it."

I chose a new gynecologist. But not by using physician referrals and checking medical directories as I would have before, when I thought I was sophisticated. "Is your gynecologist a nice person?" I asked friends. "Are you treated with dignity and consideration? Called by your first name or your last?" Another survey with few surprises. Not many women answered "yes," "yes," and "last name."

But some did. (And yes, my new gynecologist is board-certified, as nearly everyone in a metropolitan area seems to be these days.) So far, so good, but next Friday both of us will have to pass our big tests in the operating room. Will I have malignant cells on my pelvic wall? Will he resist the temptation to say "Hi, Lucille" when I'm flat on my back and going down for the count?

Health and self-respect, I've learned, are both necessaries.

# THE MARK OF A SURVIVOR

## David Yost, M.D.

It was 11:30 on a Friday night, and the emergency department patient board had been continuously full since noon. Thirty more minutes remained in my shift, with the endless flow of wheezing, abdominal discomfort, chest pain, and lacerations. I found myself becoming increasingly adept at the rapid and efficient movement of patients through the department: a five-minute history, a four-minute physical, then the necessary lab and radiological workup and they were on the way to the appropriate therapy, inpatient service, or follow-up clinic.

A new name appeared on the board for a room in which the housekeeper's mop marks had barely dried. The black wax pencil letters read "69 y.o. M with known metastatic lung CA—new onset SOB & pedal edema."

"I got a call on this guy a short while ago," my attending said quietly. "It sounds like a pretty definite medicine admit. Get the basics on him and we'll try to get him upstairs as soon as possible."

The sight was not entirely unexpected. The bed contained a thin, still man with only a few wisps of fine red hair left after extensive radiation therapy. Sunken eyes stared blankly at my nametag. The weight on the chart read "90 lbs" where one might have expected 150 for his stature. His speech was slow and halting as he struggled to answer the obligatory questions of date, place, and events of the past

week. The weary couple who had accompanied him handed
me a copy of his previous records, which indicated the cancer had recently invaded his brain and liver. I proceeded
methodically with the physical examination while acquiring
a few more key history points from the two family members. I scrawled the highlights on the chart as they talked
and the patient lay silent: "Increased JVD, diffuse basilar
rales bilaterally, regular cardiac rate and rhythm without
murmurs, 2+ pitting edema." I had already written "skin—
negative" when I noticed the small string of tattooed letters
and numbers on his left forearm.

"Where did you get this?" I asked, fully expecting yet
another blank look or some faltering words and preparing
to turn to the family members for the irrelevant answer.

"Auschwitz." The word from the man on the bed was
clear and strong. "It is the mark of one who survived," he
said steadily, with his eyes now focused intently on mine. I
turned to his family and they silently nodded.

A man who only minutes before could not clearly recall
his symptoms of the past few days now spoke with unfal-
tering precision of life events of more than 40 years ago. I
leaned against the cold wall and listened. Thirty minutes
later I left the room knowing someone who had survived
the worst of times, a man whose current physique was robust in comparison with the 70-lb frame that had survived
months of imprisonment in several concentration camps. As
part of that experience, he had participated in an 18-day
starvation march of 1500 men from the Buchenwald camp.
As one of the 300 to be alive on the 18th day, he then faced
the fire of machine guns in a massacre of those remaining.
A man who lived only by feigning death beneath the pile of
bodies and garbage, he repeatedly told me, "I am alive
because I was strong. I learned to hide, to run, and to fight.
I learned not to give up."

His adamant words and gaze would not leave me as I
stared at the enormous mediastinal mass on his chest film.

"Looks like he's not going to get away from this one,"
remarked the radiology resident as the films rolled by. My

training told me this was true, but I felt unworthy to explain to my patient that he was quickly becoming the loser in this last fight.

Shift change had come and gone during my time with him, and I carefully signed him over to the house officer taking my place. The facts were presented precisely; his condition was outlined well.

"Anything else I should know about him?" my replacement asked. I knew there was more, but I was at a loss to reconvey justly the story I had heard.

"Yeah," I said, heading toward the locker room. "If you have a few minutes, ask him about his tattoo."

# MESSAGES

## Jane A. McAdams, M.D.

Perhaps the fact that the Great Depression hit just as she and my father were starting out to raise their family had something to do with it. But no matter. Already as a small child I was aware that in the handling of money my mother was more than simply thrifty; she was downright frugal. Extravagances and luxuries did not exist. She never bought anything, for example, unless she was certain she would use it. And not only use it, but use it to the best purpose and for the longest possible time. The one exception was a new, frilly, never-worn nightgown that she kept in the bottom drawer of the bureau. But even that had its purpose: "In case I should ever have to go into the hospital," she said.

And so the nightgown lay there for years, carefully protected in its tissue wrappings.

But one day, many years later, the time came. The nightgown with its now yellowed lace and limp ruffles was taken from its wrappings and my mother entered the hospital, seeking an answer to the mysterious fevers, sweats, and malaise that had plagued her like a flu since autumn. The time was early January, in the deepest, darkest days of a cold winter, just before her 69th birthday.

We did not have long to wait for an answer. It came with the finality of a period at the end of a long sentence of strung-out clauses: lymphoma, disseminated, progressive. Privately, her physician told me he was sorry, there was probably only a matter of two or three weeks left, certainly less than even a month.

For days, I agonized over what to do with this information that only I had been told. Should I tell the family? Should I tell my mother? Did she already know? If not, did she suspect? Surely she must after so many months of malaise. Could I talk about it with her? Could I give her any hope? Could I keep up any hope she might have? Was there in fact any hope?

Some relief came when I realized her birthday was approaching. The nightgown she had saved all those years she was now wearing, but it was hopelessly dated. I resolved to lift her spirits by buying her the handsomest and most expensive matching nightgown and robe I could find. If I could not hope to cure her disease, at least I could make her feel like the prettiest patient in the entire hospital.

For a long time after she unwrapped her birthday present, given early so she would have longer to enjoy it, my mother said nothing. Finally she spoke. "Would you mind," she said, pointing to the wrapping and gown spread across the bed, "returning it to the store? I don't really want it." Then she picked up the newspaper and turned to the last page. "This is what I really want, if you could get that," she said. What she pointed to was a display advertisement of expensive designer summer purses.

My reaction was one of disbelief. Why would my mother, so careful about extravagances, want an expensive summer purse in January, one that she could not possibly use until June? She would not even live until spring, let alone summer. Almost immediately, I was ashamed and appalled at my clumsiness, ignorance, insensitivity, call it what you will. With a shock, I realized she was finally asking me what I thought about her illness. She was asking me how long she would live. She was, in fact, asking me if I thought she would live even six months. And she was telling me that if I showed I believed she would live until then, then she would do it. She would not let that expensive purse go unused. That day, I returned the gown and robe and bought the summer purse.

That was many years ago. The purse is worn out and long gone, as are at least half a dozen others. And next week my mother flies to California to celebrate her 83rd birthday. My gift to her? The most expensive designer purse I could find. She'll use it well.

*The practice of medicine has always been associated with* the laying on of hands. *Long ago, the tribal healer, limited in his therapeutic options, moistened a fevered brow or gave a comforting touch. Only later did these early practitioners discover that it was possible to discern the cause of a sickness by putting their hands on a patient's body.*

*Certain diseases were soon known to cause the heart to beat in a different rhythm, either faster or slower or in an irregular fashion. This change in the normal state of the body's "pump" could be detected by holding a patient's wrist and feeling the character of the pulse. Other illnesses would produce warmth or swelling in certain parts of the body, and a gentle laying on of hands could lead to a specific diagnosis. Hands could heal, too, not just by putting a poultice over a wound or setting a broken bone, but it seemed that the mere touch of another's hands often brought about an improvement.*

*Despite today's technological marvels such as CT scanners and magnetic resonance imagers that allow doctors to peer inside a patient's chest, abdomen, or skull, physicians still use their hands as the primary tools for exploration of the body. We use the term* palpation *to describe what doctors are doing when their fingers and hands search out the normal contours of body organs or probe the shape of an abnormality. When they tap one hand laid upon the body with another, feeling and listening for changes in resonance in the normal sounds of air- or fluid-filled cavities such as the lungs or abdomen, it's called* percussion.

*Some say that modern machinery and microchips have supplanted the usefulness of these time-honored maneuvers, but no one doubts the unique ability to comfort that is relegated to the touch of another person. In fact recent studies have shown that premature babies who are fondled and massaged by their nurses in the intensive care unit do better than infants left alone.*

*The very word* touch *itself is inextricably linked with our emotions. When someone is affected or moved by an emotional experience we say that he or she was* touched *by it. The tear-jerking end to* Terms of Endearment *or* Brian's Song *brings about an emotional response, and we call it a* touching *moment. As a matter of fact, when we speak of an emotional state we use the term* feeling, *and the universal greeting of* how are you *is synonymous with* how do you feel.

*It is curious that the Latin word* manus *meaning hand is so close to what we call ourselves as a species. Certainly many of our words used to describe emotion are about our hands. When we speak of powerfully changing or controlling another person, we use the word* manipulation, *and when a difficult emotional situation arises, we tell others that we can* manage *or* handle *it. We join hands in prayer, in the bond of marriage, and in greeting each other. It is no surprise, then, that we also speak of healing hands. Clearly it is our hands that make us human.*

*Since it was first published, I've read the next essay more than 50 times, often aloud to friends. Each time I've thought about the vital importance of touching and comforting another human being. And after each reading, I've had to wipe my eyes.*

B.B.D.

# THE MUSIC AND THE MEDICINE

## Elizabeth D. Vickers

The harmonica sticking out of his lab coat pocket suggested that an unusual physician was walking into the hospital examining room. His slightly stooped shoulders made his 6-ft frame appear slightly shorter, and the hairline of his brown, curly hair, flecked with gray, was receding. Heavy, black-and-silver-rimmed glasses framed his green eyes, and the scars of teenage acne and the wrinkles of 50 years lined his face. The breast pocket of his stiffly starched white coat bulged with an assortment of pens and pencils, a penlight, several tongue blades, and the harmonica. As he greeted the elderly lady on the examining table, his hands commanded attention. Their wide span dwarfed the patient's in a firm but reassuring handshake. Huge veins were outlined on the backs of these hairy hands. The fingernails were clean and clipped short. As he asked her how she felt, he discreetly pulled down the sheet, lifted her gown, and gently palpated her abdomen. She replied she was much better but he suspected differently; his hands felt the tumor. He carefully pulled up the sheet and quietly described the examination he was going to do. She would swallow a flexible tube about the size of her middle finger. It would enable him to see into her stomach. Medicine would be injected into her vein so she would be drowsy and relaxed, but he believed that music was the best relaxant. As he slowly reached for his har-

monica, he asked for her favorite tune. She blushed and
said that she was from the country and only knew gospel
songs. He handled the harmonica as if it were fine porce-
lain. She touched his arm and asked if he knew "Will the
Circle Be Unbroken?" He raised the harmonica to his lips,
cupped it with his hands, and brought the strains of the
old hymn from the harp. The music and the medicine
seeped into the elderly woman. When she began to breathe
heavily, he returned the harmonica to his pocket and proceeded with the examination.

# A MEDICAL STUDENT ON CALL

## Adria Burrows

It was the first night on call of my medicine rotation and
my intern handed me a couple of tubes and told me to draw
blood from Mrs. Matthews, a patient with advanced glioblastoma multiforme.

Her room was dim, lighted only by a streetlamp outside.
I could see her shaved head and obese body, a huge mound
under the sheets. Her wrists were tied to the bed at her
sides. Snoring loudly, mouth half open, she lay on her
back, and I shook her shoulder gently and called out her
name, but the snores continued. Nevertheless, I talked to
her, mostly because I was nervous on the second day of my
new rotation and I felt like talking to someone.

"Hello, Mrs. Matthews," I said. "I just want to get
some blood from you. This will just take a few minutes
and then you can go back to sleep." The snoring stopped,

but otherwise there was no sign of waking. I took one of her huge arms and began to draw the blood. "It's raining outside, so you're not missing much out there, Mrs. Matthews," I went on. "Hold your arm still. I just need a little more blood and then I'll be done. You're a real trooper. All done. Thank you." Her short arm had large purple splotches on it: obviously many people had taken blood from her before. As I left the room, her snores resumed.

I began to take blood from Mrs. Matthews every day and kept talking to her as I would to my conscious patients, just in case she did hear me. She would stop snoring when I spoke to her, which was sign enough to me that she might be listening. So each day as I took some blood, I gave her the weather report, told her that her hair was starting to grow in on her head nicely, and sometimes would even tell her of a lecture I had attended.

One day I walked in to find that Mrs. Matthews' eyes were open and she was watching me. I tried to picture her with a full head of hair and some lipstick and actually saw a very pretty 60-year-old woman. I greeted her as I usually did, but she soon closed her eyes. I was disappointed, but went on talking anyway, saying that she had beautiful eyes that looked like my mother's.

Last night I needed blood from Mrs. Matthews and she was snoring again, but her face was less pale. Her hair was bristly and her puffy cheeks shook as she breathed. I gave her my usual hello, took her arm, and had begun to give her the weather report when she opened her eyes suddenly and her lips began to quiver.

"What is it, Mrs. Matthews, are you in pain?" I asked. She raised her head from the pillow slightly, and I bent closer to her.

"I—I—" she began. I waited. "You—you talked to me. The others—they thought I was fat and—ugly. That I was dead. Couldn't hear." Her head collapsed back onto the pillow. "Not you. You talked and I heard." She closed her eyes and began to snore again, but her huge hand reached out for something. I instinctively took it, and she squeezed my hand with surprising strength. Her eyelids quivered and she mumbled in her sleeplike state. Then her hand loosened, as though she were exhausted from the effort.

After I had her blood, I patted her on the hand and thanked her for speaking to me. She went on snoring, her eyes still closed. I turned out the light and said good-night. I closed the door for the night and made my way to the lab, my hand still aching from the sharp squeeze.

# THE LIE

## Lawrence D. Grouse, M.D., Ph.D.

Annie is from New Hampshire and came here to the foothills of the Blue Ridge Mountains for the horse show. The nurses and I carry her from the car into the emergency room and gently place her on the gurney. She was kicked in the abdomen by her horse and lay in a field for over an hour until friends found her and brought her to the hospital. Even though I am working in the emergency room of a small hospital, I am confident. The nurses know their jobs. Faced with a serious surgical problem, we work well together.

Within a few minutes we have inserted two IVs, one in a forearm vein, another in the external jugular; her blood pressure, however, remains marginal. The fluid from the abdominal tap is grossly bloody and so is her urine. Annie remains calm. Her serious eyes are piercing; I hold her hand to reassure her, but also to take her pulse. She is bleeding very rapidly into her abdomen. Nothing I do seems to help, and I am scared. She is in shock, yet she converses politely and inquires about her condition.

"Thank you for helping me," she says. "Really, it wasn't the horse's fault!"

"We're not worried about the horse, Annie," I say. "The horse is fine."

"Is it a serious injury?" She pauses. "Will I live?"

"Everything will work out, Annie," I tell her. "It may be a little rough for a bit, but it will work out."

"Are you sure?" she asks, gazing steadily at me. "Please, tell me honestly."

I don't answer for a moment. I look at her. I am already fond of her and I do not want to lie. I squeeze her hand and smile. I am unsure how she will do, but I say, "Yes, I'm sure."

After a third IV is in place, her blood pressure stabilizes. The general surgeon and the urologist arrive and plan their emergency workup and exploratory surgery. I breathe a sigh of relief as they take charge of her care. Suddenly, we find that the door to the surgical suite in the emergency room has been inadvertently locked and the head nurse's key won't open it. Annie and a nurse are locked inside. There is a great deal of key rattling and doorknob shaking. The pitch of people's voices starts to rise. I break into a sweat. The head nurse yells orders into the telephone and almost immediately three burly maintenance men with crowbars appear.

"Get rid of that door! Now!" the head nurse bellows.

The door is splintered in 20 seconds. Annie is laughing, tells us not to worry, tells us that she is fine. She thinks it is the funniest scene ever.

At surgery, we find that Annie has a severely lacerated liver and a ruptured kidney. The liver is repaired; the kidney is removed, but when I wake up the next morning and look in on Annie, disseminated intravascular coagulation has developed and she is receiving heparin. Four nurses and two physicians have already given blood for her. The intensive

care unit hosts a steady stream of staff who have helped
Annie and who come by with a few encouraging words. Her
parents have arrived. Annie's father is a college professor:
a tall, angular man, feeling frightened and out of place.
Annie's mother is a small woman with delicate features. The
surgeon's wife accompanies them. By the following day,
when I leave the hospital after my weekend shift, several of
the staff, including the head nurse, have each given two
units of blood for Annie.

Two weeks later—during my next shift—I am waylaid and
hugged by a happy and ambulatory Annie.

"Everyone here has been so good to me," Annie beams.

As we sit over a cup of coffee, her parents timidly inquire
whether Annie might have been close to death on her arrival
at the hospital. I can't help bragging about treating Annie
in the emergency room. As I launch into the story, I find
that Annie remembers it all, and she chimes in with an exact
rendition of our entire conversation on the day of the accident. I am amazed! She was in shock, and still she remembers every word I said. I finish my story with a flourish.
"When I found that you had abdominal bleeding and I still
couldn't bring up your blood pressure with two IVs, I have
to admit that I thought you were a goner."

Annie seems shocked to hear this. She looks at me angrily and says, "Don't you remember? You said you were
sure I would live. I remembered that promise all the time!
I put a great deal of weight on what you said, and you . . ."
Suddenly, for the first time since the accident, and to everyone's surprise, tears are in her eyes and she is weeping; she
is inconsolable because I lied to her.

# Sudden Intimacies

## Michael Radetsky, M.D., C.M.

For over a year this infant had spent more of his time in the hospital than out. He had a form of histiocytosis X with immunodeficiency, but no one truly knew the prognosis. We had all hoped for the best: that he would slowly outgrow his disease while we treated the interminable complications as they arose. He was a darling boy, with a round face, a willing smile, his father's tendency to crinkle up his nose, and blond hair that stood up vertically on his head. He was readmitted to the hospital because his fever had returned and the eczematous rash had flared up. None of us thought that he would die. But, he developed a right-sided facial palsy, began to choke on his secretions, and had to be intubated. Seizures followed, with coma and eventual brain death due to uncertain causes.

One week before the boy's death, his father brought in a new toy, a stuffed dinosaur emblazoned with swirls of color. As was customary with him, the father began to brandish the animal in order to evoke some flicker of interest from his comatose son. "Hey, bud, look! A dinosaur! Hey, look at it!" Nothing happened. Then, the boy's one good eye opened slightly and fixed on the brightly colored animal prancing so close to his face. A small smile tugged at the left corner of his mouth, and slowly his right arm reached out to embrace the toy. Within a minute, the smile faded,

24

and the boy lapsed back into coma. We all cried. He died the following week without regaining consciousness.

What fulfills the physician? Certainly, the diagnostic challenge, the financial security, the altruistic glow, and the grateful thanks all provide a measure of satisfaction. But all too often, success becomes bracketed by failure, a deluge of new information erodes the sense of professional mastery, money ceases to compensate fully for the time and toil, the good one attempts to do goes awry, and the thankfulness of patients becomes admixed with fear and suspicion.

No, for me fulfillment comes from the sudden intimacies with total strangers—those moments when the human barrier cracks open to reveal what is most secret and inarticulate. A word can betray the deepest emotion. A look can reflect a world of feeling. Illness strips away superficiality to reveal reality in etched detail. This revelation can fuse together disparate lives in unexpected kinship. Is it the fear of death, the dreaded pain, the sorrow, or the loss? The physician who can see is there to share in it. Is the joy of birth, of unforeseen recovery, of reunion with one considered lost? The physician who cares can rejoice even as a family member. Who else so often listens to the whispered thought, holds the hand, puzzles over the vagaries of fate, and feels another's moment so personally and powerfully? And who else has such a chance to realize that it matters less whether a moment is one of supreme sadness or supreme joy than it does that the moment itself is supreme?

This is the physician's privilege: to be lifted out of the dross of common days in order to experience such clarity of feeling. The intensity of birth and death, pleasure and sorrow as expressed in the lives of others has the power to nullify personal boundaries in sudden communion. Then, the world is seen in its proper proportions, and the tenuous miracle of existence is underscored. Surely it must profit us to feel this deeply, with the hope that somehow, in the sweep of that feeling, we might yet learn to appreciate the wondrous happening of our own lives.

# 'ALONELY'

## Lawrence D. Grouse, M.D., Ph.D.

During the first semester of her freshman year at a liberal arts college in New York City, Allison got pregnant. Her boyfriend, who was the captain of a student rugby team, refused to see her until the pregnancy was terminated, but he reassured her that everything between them would be fine after the abortion. Allison's family took the same stance as her boyfriend, but their plan was not acceptable to Allison. Instead, she left school and moved in with her 76-year-old grandmother, Mrs. Simpson, who lived alone in a ramshackle townhouse in south Baltimore.

Allison insisted on being self-supporting; she found a job in the collections department of a building supply company. When Cassandra was born, Allison missed only two days of work. The grandmother did her best to cope with the baby during the day, but she was hard of hearing and she always seemed very tired. At night Allison cried whenever she was reminded that, because of her job, she had not been able to breast-feed her baby.

Tony was a swashbuckler; his extravagant plans and passions attracted Allison. His comfortable way of life in spite of no visible means of support seemed to her a remarkable achievement. Most important, Tony told her that he wanted to legally adopt Cassandra. They were married over a three-day weekend. It was not until after the marriage that she realized that the majority of his income came from selling

26

marijuana. For two years they lived in a run-down apartment complex called the Camino Real. Allison continued to work at the building supply company, and it became Tony's job to watch Cassandra during the day. Allison did the remainder of the child care as well as the cooking, laundry, and housekeeping. She never mentioned to him that her income was their principal source of support. At the Camino Real she grew accustomed to hearing muffled curses and shattering furniture as well as the sounds of blows landing on human skin.

When Cassandra was 2 years old, Allison became concerned about her. Whenever she would come home unexpectedly she would find Cassandra sitting in her crib while Tony would be lying on the couch watching television or not in the apartment at all. The marriage ended abruptly one night when Allison came home to find Cassandra soiled, hungry, and shivering in her crib. Her eyes were tightly shut and she was desperately sucking her finger in the dark. Tony had passed out on the couch. First, Allison ejected him from the apartment. Then she threw all his belongings into the hallway. When they were alone she rocked Cassandra until she finally opened her eyes. The child kept repeating, "I want to be alonely!"

I took care of Mrs. Simpson when she had a bout with pneumonia, and as a result I became Allison and Cassandra's physician as well. My first impression of the child was that she was like a dark angel; she had sloe eyes, an olive complexion, and long black hair. Cassandra insisted on having fingernail polish just like her mother, and I noticed that the polish was always absent from the index finger of her right hand. Her moods were mercurial. Other than a few ear infections and an accidental ingestion of a small amount of household bleach the previous year, there had been no medical problems. Most important, her development was on schedule for a 4-year-old. Allison remained apprehensive about the effects of Cassandra's unsettled infancy, but nothing that I saw indicated any long-lasting developmental disruption.

Once, after Allison and Cassandra had left the office, I asked the nurse what she thought about Allison's insistence on having and raising a child by herself and how it might affect the child.

"There's no understanding fanatics!" she said with a vehemence that surprised me.

Often when Cassandra came into the office with an illness she kept repeating, almost like a chant, "I want to be alonely! I want to be alonely!" I asked Allison what this meant, and she told me that she had always assumed it just meant that Cassandra was sad and wanted to be alone. It had been one of her first sentences. It was poignant and even humorous to see Cassandra with her eyes tightly shut, chanting, "I want to be alonely!" I wondered what she meant by "alonely." It didn't seem to me that she really wanted to be either "alone" or "lonely." It always unsettled me to see her disconsolate even though I knew that after the shot or the ear infection was over the sadness would be gone and her smile would return.

Practicing in a small town near Baltimore meant that I saw my patients at the grocery store or mowing their lawns more frequently than I saw them in the office. I liked this about my practice. It also meant that a death touched me and had an effect on the practice more than it might have in some other settings. When Mrs. Simpson died of a heart attack I was among those gathered at the funeral home. Allison was also there and she was visibly shaken, but Cassandra was composed. Some of the people present, I noticed, immediately wept when they viewed the body. Others seated themselves and wept quietly after a thoughtful pause.

Allison and Cassandra spoke to no one at the funeral home. Their isolation was painfully obvious, and afterward when Allison asked me if they could ride with me to the cemetery I was happy to oblige. During the drive Allison seemed drained and forlorn, but Cassandra was excited and preoccupied. She asked her mother, "Who lives in all the houses when the people die?" This question was too much for Allison, so I tried to make a diplomatic answer. Cassandra then asked her mother where Grandmother was going. Allison haltingly explained, "She is going to be with God." Cassandra wanted to pursue this point but saw that she should not. It was stiflingly hot at the cemetery, and mosquitoes were everywhere. During the eulogy at the grave site, Cassandra kept looking intently at each of the mourners. She finally whispered to me, "Which one is God?"

As I drove them home, Cassandra asked a stream of questions about death, which I tried to answer without further upsetting Allison. This effort was unsuccessful. Allison covered her eyes and began to cry. The child couldn't understand why her mother was so upset, and she grew impatient with her.

"Mommy, you don't have to cry any more!" she said. "Grandma is alonely now!"

*The death of another person is a circumstance that most of us have to face only a few times in our lives. The vast majority of people rarely think about dying, and when they do it's usually in the abstract. But doctors are steeped in sickness, 24 hours a day. Most people may think about disease only a few times in their lives when they are ill, but doctors are surrounded by disease every day.*

*How can doctors come home from work each day and have a normal life if the preceding 12 hours were filled with the sorrow of others? Most attempt to protect themselves and their families from the tragedies that suffuse their lives. Some distance themselves from the emotional turmoil and seem to be almost isolated, appearing perhaps cold and callous. Others do not fare so well; physician suicide and alcohol and drug abuse may stem in part from the constant emotional bombardment.*

*Most find another way out—in humor. Granted, the humor is often bizarre, a sort of "gallows" humor, but it is exactly that sense of the macabre that is necessary to fend off the realities of what they face each and every day. The lurid and ghastly comedy so often seen in M\*A\*S\*H and St. Elsewhere is an attempt to deal with the all too real aspects of medicine.*

*I spent almost a decade of my life living in a hospital. I slept and dreamed while encircled by the restless nights of others. I ate my meals surrounded by those getting their sustenance from plastic tubes inserted in their veins. I walked into rooms from which others would never leave. I worked and I played and I spent most of my days in a place where most people are frightened to go.*

*How do you deal with it? Most of the time you just have to laugh.*

B. B. D.

# MILESTONES

## Gary A. Chinman

### I.

He was the first patient assigned to me on my medicine rotation. I met him on the first day. He was the first person I ever drew blood from, the first I ever started an IV on. And he was my first patient ever to die.

Mr. Sweeney was a robust man. He was a bulldozer-backhoe driver and mechanic and he looked it. At 62 he had a muscular upper body, thick toughened hands, and a 50s-type crewcut, although Mr. Sweeney, I'm sure, never tried to be stylish. He was thoughtfully honest in answering my questions in a hoarse Marlon Brando voice and an easy, sometimes sheepish smile.

He seemed like a nice guy, a real Vermonter, taciturn and uncomplaining. He also seemed puzzled to find himself in the hospital and confused by the doctors' serious words. Most of all he seemed perplexed by the cancer that was destroying his liver. A few weeks earlier he had been an apparently healthy man. Now his belly bulged with a liver the size of a volleyball, causing him the kind of pain only narcotics could touch. The doctors spoke of chemotherapy and resuscitation orders: Would he want CPR, the paddles, life on a respirator? He didn't seem to understand; he talked of wanting a bowel movement.

Published data told me Mr. Sweeney would, in fact, soon

die. His oncologist was optimistic about the upcoming chemo.

"What'll it give him?" I asked. "A year and a half?"

"Not that long," he said. "More like a year."

*"Just one year?"* And for that, I thought, we give him poisons until he's continuously nauseated. Why don't we just give him pain meds and let him die at home?

I felt especially frustrated the day I needed five tubes of blood and clumsily stuck him six times because of my lack of skill. His face registered such stoic dismay that I quickly apologized.

"That's OK," he rasped. "Let's get it over with."

I *tried* to get it over with but by the time I was done he had ugly bruises on each arm and lay in bed with his palms up and eyes closed like a suppliant asking why. I jabbered another apology and slunk out of the room, angry at the regimen that made me do this to him.

Our chemotherapy did not help Mr. Sweeney. Instead it pushed him over the edge by damaging his remaining few healthy liver cells: after one treatment he became jaundiced and nearly comatose. He pulled through but never returned to his admission baseline. After 21 days his arms were broomsticks, his voice was gone, and his face was grayish yellow, with deep eye sockets and concave cheeks. His breathing was labored and ugly-sounding as if his lungs were full of muck. And the next afternoon, while I was in the next room drawing blood (successfully this time) on another patient, Mr. Sweeney died.

I'm convinced there is a series of milestones one passes during this process of medical education. The first is joyfully reading and rereading that initial letter of acceptance. The next is those year 1 midterms. After that it's probably getting past part 1 of the boards. And next is watching your first patient die. Like any real milestone it demarcates entry into a new realm where the territory is suddenly different and the traveler somehow changed. I still want to be a physician and, now more than ever, I want to be the most effective physician I can be. I don't think I have any illusions about potentially being able to save everyone. I just want to make a difference in my patients' lives. And in their deaths.

## II.

Four days after Mr. Sweeney died, I sat at the hospital's computer terminal to get my patients' lab data. I was especially interested in Tom Leclerc's values, since he was my favorite patient at the time, a sweet old guy who always seemed to underplay his suffering. I punched up his number and the computer gave me an uncooperative beep.

"Oh come on," I mumbled, remembering that the system was newly installed. I tried the same numbers.

Beep, went the machine, with no other information.

"Jeez, what's going on?" I wondered. The only other times this happened was when the patient had left the hospital, either by discharge or . . . I turned to the student next to me.

"Tony, anybody die last night?"

"Uh, let me think. Yeah, just one. One guy."

"Tom Leclerc," I blurted. "Was it Tom Leclerc?"

"Yeah, that's right. That's who it was."

"Tom Leclerc *died*? Are you sure?"

"Yes, Gary, I'm sure. I'm sorry."

"Oh, shit," I whispered. *"Dammit."*

The previous evening I had sat on Tom's bed discussing his cancer. He knew he was in bad shape but just wanted to make it to his 73rd birthday, six weeks hence. No problem, I had said. And I sincerely meant it. After all, he had done this chemo bit before with no complications and he had come in this time smiling and talkative, just five days earlier. I steered the conversation to his not eating for three days.

"We gotta get some food inside you," I had said. "You'll feel better."

"Yeah, but I hate the food here," he had said. "Even the

smell makes me sick. Y'know, the last time I was in here I got all my food across the street, at HoJo's.''

Actually, I had already known this and was ready.

"You like HoJo's burgers? Would you drink a milk shake?''

"I'd try."

"OK, I'll be back in a minute with your dinner. But you gotta promise me you'll eat it."

"I'll try," he smiled.

When I returned with the food, Tom seemed to perk up. As I left he was happily opening the Styrofoam take-out box.

That was the last time I saw him.

I remembered all this the next morning. I was stunned. I walked the halls briefly, pulling myself together. I saw my other patients, then joined my team at the weekly morbidity and mortality conference. I sat next to my resident, a very competent doc with a good sense of humor.

"Tom Leclerc died last night," I whispered.

"Yeah, I heard," he said.

Then he paused, looked me in the eye, and said with a completely deadpan expression: "Last time *I* eat at Ho-Jo's."

I couldn't help it. I had to laugh.

# NUMBER 46

## Russell Portenoy, M.D.

She was billed as a cord compression. A streetwise woman with intuitive grasp and a likely lump of cancer in her spine. He was admitting resident for the day. He placed the telephone back in its cradle after hearing the story and screwed up his face in a typical spasm of fatigued distaste. The ones with cancer were so draining and the cords were probably the worst of these. There were always more tests to order, consultations to arrange, explanations to give and give again. He opened a book and waited for the floor to call him.

She was wearing a yellow robe with the collar buttoned high on her neck. He asked his routine history questions. She called him "Doctor" and paused after every question, assuming it had importance beyond the apparent and wanting the answers to be precise. Every so often her chin would quiver, and she would close her mouth and purse her lips to quell the movement. As she lifted her hands from her knees to her body and drew a line to where the tingling had ascended and stopped, her eyelids rose and the dark pupils were framed in desperate white.

He fidgeted some and allowed part of himself to consider other things. "Ever shoot up?"

She shook her head. "Not for me, Doctor."

"Any violence to your back?"

Her tone captured his disappointment. "I've been mostly in bed."

"Any TB?"

She lifted her head and her eyes widened further. "My man was quarantined for that last year. But the skin test they gave my kids and me at that time didn't show anything."

He nodded slowly and met her eyes. A vivid memory seeped into his mind. A wrinkled old man sat on a bed like this one. He spoke in a brogue and flashed an easy grin, a badge of indestructibility, exuding health. The seizures in his arm were sure to be an old vascular nothing. The man was reassured; his children shook the doctor's hand as if the choice of the lesion was his. Sometime later his case was presented at conference. The radiologist snorted smugly as he pointed out the deadly rings of white on the scan. It was no surprise to him that so many metastases could hide in such a capacious skull. The clinical exam is crude, he reminded the crowd.

The first set of films was done late that night. He peered at them alone at a viewbox in an empty corridor. A novice, he eschewed the gestalt and catalogued the abnormalities. The mass extended beyond the spine and had abolished the normal architecture, scarring the bone and obliterating the disk. Could it be infection? As the minutes passed, the shadows seemed to become less uncertain. "Number one, infection," he mumbled to himself, "a distant second, cancer."

He stopped by her room. She was awake, staring blankly at a television with its volume turned too low to hear. The terror in her large dark eyes bounced back at him and he smiled with false confidence, tapping her reflexes and scratching the bottom of her feet.

"I feel optimistic about you," he said. "Tumor's possible, but it looks good for infection."

"Please, God."

He smiled again. "It looks very good for infection."

The films he had seen were hanging neatly beside the myelogram when he met with the radiologist the next morning. The older man called for the ones in training and waited for a group to gather. "You almost didn't need a myelogram in this case," he began, squinting at the zone of the destruction and cupping his hands around it as if framing for a portrait. "The pattern is clear here. Number one, lymphoma; number two, metastases."

"Could it be infection?" he asked softly.

The radiologist grinned. "Number 46."

Preparations were made for surgery. There seemed always to be another test to order, another consultation to obtain. He measured the weakness in her legs and ran a pin up her back to find progression. Stoically, she signed the consent for operation. It didn't seem the time for long explanations.

He returned to start her intravenous line. As the needle pierced her skin, he caught the quiver in her chin and the movement of her lips to halt it.

"What do you think it is?" she asked him.

He shrugged and adjusted the flow from the bottle at her bedside. "We hope it's infection."

Gently she closed her eyes and swallowed, her quivering lips pressed tightly together. "There's no way to tell which?"

He woodenly added a piece of tape to the uneven square of white on her wrist. "There's no bad news yet."

The corners of her mouth twitched upward and she lifted her head toward the bland religious print that hung above her bed. "It's worse not knowing." A tear broke free and meandered down her cheek. "I can't prepare myself."

He felt exposed, unbalanced, the rules of the game they were playing switched abruptly midway. His head dropped and he reached forward to lay a hand on her arm. "The most likely thing is cancer. I think you have a kind of cancer."

She wiped her face with her knuckles and nodded. Her mouth twisted into a grim smile and there passed a long and unsteady silence. "Thank you, Doctor," she said finally.

The next day the word circulated quickly. Her films were copied for the teaching file and the student on Infectious

Disease came to read her chart for a presentation. The radiologist made ill-tempered grunting sounds and the surgeon could be heard expounding eloquently on that great mimic, tuberculosis.

He heard the news when she was in the recovery room. She was wiggling her toes, he was told, and the tingling was already gone. He felt the strength leave him like water from a ruptured pipe. He made his excuses. Suddenly, he wanted to be alone.

# Not on My Shift

## Lynn A. Crosby, M.D.

She was a 72-year-old woman who had been recently transferred by helicopter from a smaller hospital. She had started bleeding from a duodenal ulcer and was in serious condition. The attending surgeon and medical consultant both agreed to try aggressive medical management because of the risks of surgery. But she continued to bleed despite treatment and was taken to surgery that evening.

It was a Saturday night, and I was getting a report from the surgical resident who had been on call the previous shift. "We had quite a time with your patient last night," he said. "She survived the operation, but I think she'll probably die sometime today."

"Not on my shift," I blurted out without thinking.

As I went through my surgical rotation in medical school, and now in residency, this situation had come up many times. There was always one patient on a service who was close to death. The residents did everything possible not to let the patient die on their night on call. It was inevitable that the patient would die, but to let that person die on your shift was a sign of failure.

My night on call started as usual: an admission from the emergency room to rule out appendicitis, a traffic accident victim with only superficial wounds, a few calls to the floor. Then I was called to the intensive care unit. My patient's blood pressure was dropping, and her urine output was low. From that point, I was in and out of the ICU all night: increasing her fluids, transfusing blood, adding a dopamine drip, inserting a catheter and an arterial line, giving albumin, putting her on a ventilator; it went on and on.

Finally, it was 7 AM, time for me to give the report to the next surgical resident. I described the evening's work with my patient and said that she was in serious condition, that I thought she would probably die during the day.

The oncoming surgical resident flashed back, "Not on my shift!"

# THE TALLIS CASE

## David T. Nash, M.D.

I approach my responsibilities of teaching cardiology to medical students and house officers with some ambivalence. Of course, I have always enjoyed and usually learned something from my contacts with these young colleagues, but lately their emphasis seems to be entirely on technical procedures. Few of my charges express an interest in entering full-time solo practice; most are not enthusiastic about honing their skills in bedside physical diagnosis. None believes in house calls.

I can remember making house calls on people who were too poor for a society doctor but too proud for the clinic. My mind can still conjure up the kind of call I'd get, almost always at night.

"Doctor, can you come? Quick! It's Zadhr, he's not feeling too good."

"What seems to be the trouble?"

"How should I know? He just doesn't feel good. Please come."

It was usually more a plea than a command. I'd roll over to the side of the bed and fall into my clothes. Bleary-eyed, I'd stagger to my car and fume because it started so slowly in the cold. Heated garages were an unachieved luxury when I started in practice. Somehow I'd find the address, although more often than not I'd get lost in the process. About the time I was cursing under my breath, I'd spot the telltale light and an anxious kerchief-clad face at the window, one hand pulling the curtains apart for a better view.

"You're the doctor?" would be the greeting, punctuated by lifted eyebrows and a faint grimace of disbelief. I looked young for my age. People trusted older, more experienced doctors in those days.

"I'm Dr. Nash. Where's the patient?" I usually preferred to get right down to business, considering it was the middle of the night.

"What's your hurry? Take off your coat. Zadhr is in the bedroom." The ancient female before me was annoyed. It was obvious to her that youths no longer concerned themselves with manners, and she didn't really approve of young pishers passing themselves off as real doctors, even if one could not pay.

Her eyes spotted my little black bag and she seemed reassured for the moment. She heaved a sigh, somewhere between a grunt and a wheeze, and led the way.

The house was of typical frame construction, two-storied

and of pre-World War I vintage. The banisters that led up to the master bedroom were hand carved and glistened with a dark patina of hardwood and years of furniture polish. A threadbare runner led up the stairs. At the top I could hear the sounds of respiratory distress.

The ancient Jew sitting bolt upright in bed against several down pillows looked regal with his white beard and long sideburns. His nightclothes were white, and a small yarmulke adorned his gray, tufted scalp. Dark, bright eyes burned at me through the somber dimness of the room lit by a single 60-watt bulb. He offered no greeting or complaint, just a long soul-piercing stare. I was mesmerized for a moment, and then the noise of his breathing broke through my consciousness and I knew I had my hands full.

My physical examination was brief and confirmatory. The old man was in severe congestive heart failure. He was literally drowning in his own juices.

"Did he eat anything salty?"

"Nothing. A little schmaltz herring; a bowl of chicken soup; he doesn't eat enough."

She could not see me wince. Wisely, I stopped myself from explaining the reality of salt restriction to an old Orthodox matriarch who was salting flesh before I was born.

Well, at least I knew what had to be done.

"He has to go to the hospital. Where's the phone?"

"No!" It was the only word Zadhr had said. It did not brook discussion, but I wasn't quite wise enough to realize that.

"Look," I started, speaking a little louder than necessary to emphasize my conviction and the academic knowledge that my professors had assured me would carry the day once I got into practice. "Look, he's in heart failure. I can treat him better in the hospital. It's important."

"Doctor, you heard my husband. He doesn't want to go. Treat him here."

I knew further negotiations would be fruitless. I gave him digoxin, a diuretic, and a shot of morphine, but he was still working too hard breathing. Then my training finally came in handy. I told the old lady what I needed. With hesitation she went to the kitchen and cut the cord away from the curtains. I arranged the tourniquet around the old man's arms and legs. With the blood trapped in his extremities, he began to breathe better again.

During the next several hours, his congestive heart failure abated. Finally he dozed off, able to lie flat again for the first time in a week.

The old lady had given me several cups of tea during the long night's vigil, so I was wide awake when dawn broke. Convinced that the patient would survive, I turned to go. At the door she pressed something in my hand and murmured an awkward thanks.

As I started the engine, I opened the brown paper wrapper. Inside was a hand-embroidered tallis case, its velvet worn by a lifetime of weekly use.

I wonder how many of my students will feel as rewarded for their efforts.

# BRAD

## John D. Cantwell, M.D.

Like E.T., he is funny-looking, emits weird noises, drinks and eats whatever he gets his hands on (beer, wooden balls, plastic bananas, sponges), and brings out the best—and occasionally the worst—in those he encounters. Unlike the Extra-Terrestrial, he has a double row of teeth, repeatedly voids on his mother's best carpeting, and is not obsessed with phoning home, for he lives there, within the warmth and security of a close-knit family.

Bradley arrived on a night I was to quarterback the Mayo Clinic residents' team against a squad of Rochester construction workers (affectionately known as the "cement heads"). It was cold and rainy, a miserable night for football, so I didn't mind accompanying my wife to the labor and delivery area of St. Mary's Hospital. I was hoping for a future all-American, a Rhodes scholar, or at least an Olympic candidate.

The birth was uneventful, but within several days my tearful wife told me (a mother's intuition, I guess) that Bradley was defective. I couldn't be sure, and neither could his pediatrician. The diagnosis was finally made several months later by a 6-year-old boy in one of the waiting rooms of the Mayo Clinic:

"My, what a tiny brain," he observed, after peering at Brad for a few minutes. He was right on target, for the infant had mild microcephaly and would be severely mentally retarded and epileptic.

We moved to San Diego so I could study cardiology under Eugene Braunwald. My wife spent much of her time working with our son, feeling that it would make a great difference in his development, and expected me to do likewise. I rather resented this, as my studies were hard and my free moments all too infrequent. I didn't think my time with Brad was very productive. Once, however, when I was home alone with him, I heard gurgling sounds from his bedroom. I rushed in and found him in the midst of a grand mal seizure. When it persisted, I carried him to the car and headed for San Diego County Hospital, where I worked. En route, he became cyanotic and, shortly thereafter, stopped breathing. I administered cardiopulmonary resuscitation, as best I could under the circumstances, while racing to the emergency room. Their staff took over upon my arrival, and I was asked to sit in the waiting room. I heard a "Code 99" page and saw the cardiac arrest team dash into Brad's room. I wondered if he would make it. I had some conflicting feelings at that point, for he seemed like such a bother and had little to offer (or so I thought).

He did survive and, months later, seemed to make some progress. He would scoot along the floor after his pacifier, and we were encouraged that he was learning to crawl. We eagerly awaited our next appointment with the pediatric neurologist to show him how much Brad had improved:

"That's not really crawling," the neurologist said. "He's just making some primitive swimming-type motions on the floor." Our spirits were dashed, but received a lift when another neurologist, one a little more sensitive to people's feelings, explained:

"Yes! He really is beginning to crawl—commando-style."

We moved to Atlanta for my military service and additional cardiology training. A daughter had been born in California, and, in Georgia, another son followed. I developed a keen appreciation for their rather routine development and looked forward to spare moments when I could take them on neighborhood walks, balancing with them delicately on stone ledges and searching diligently for the troll who allegedly lived beneath the little wooden bridge in a nearby park.

Fifteen years have passed. Helped by a combined family effort and the discipline, love, and encouragement of a former nun (who directed the special school he attended), Brad has learned to walk and feed himself and has become partially toilet-trained. Through him, I discovered the Special Olympics, and soon became the "team doctor" for Georgia, complementing my other role as a team physician for the Atlanta Braves. I find similarities between both groups of athletes, namely, the importance of doing one's best with whatever abilities one has and striving always to improve.

There are light moments. A little boy inquired as to what was wrong with Brad. When told that Brad's brain didn't work real well, he advised us to take him right back to the hospital and have it fixed. The daughter of a friend kept her distance, later telling her mother that she didn't want to catch whatever it was he had. Our other children recently took a cardiopulmonary resuscitation course and were advised to put in extra time practicing on "Annie." As they explained this to me, their eyes simultaneously rested on their older brother and mischievous smiles appeared on their faces. "Don't you dare!" I admonished them. Instead, my linebacker son occasionally uses him as a tackling dummy, pouncing on him as Jack Lambert, the Steelers' ferocious player, would.

We have become accustomed to the embarrassing moments: the piercing shrieks in fast-food places, the telephone caller who asks, "Did you just get a new dog? I hear barking in the background." (No, ma'am, that's just my son.)

I no longer feel that the time I spend with Brad is wasted. On the contrary, he has become my favorite snuggling partner for weekend afternoon naps. He exudes a lot of love and tends to bring forth the best of qualities in those who encounter him. He has opened my eyes to the satisfaction of volunteer work with children like him and has brought my wife and me into a deep bond of love and understanding as we share his peaks and his valleys.

Finally, he has enhanced and matured my appreciation of his two siblings. I recall a moment when I was coaching third base in a Little League game. My younger son, a switch-hitter, came to bat, the last chance for our team to salvage an important victory. The opposing pitcher, who looked considerably older than 12 (maybe it was the mustache), was throwing bullets as the last rays of an afternoon sun gradually disappeared beneath the horizon. Ryan managed to foul off a pitch, took a called strike, and refrained from nibbling at several fast balls beyond the strike zone. I called time and discussed the situation with him. The final pitch came in at his knees. He swung hard, as I taught him to, and missed. The game was over.

I walked with him to the car, my arm around his shoulders. He can talk, he can run, and he can slide headfirst into second base like Pete Rose. I smiled, whispered a

Physicians, too, have to come to grips at least once in their lifetime with their own mortality. Doctors are so wrapped up in their patients' lives and so sure that they have control over biological processes that they often believe they are immortal. But sooner or later they, too, must face the prospect of a transient existence in this world. The prospect of my own mortality came to me during my internship.

I had been sharing the responsibility of taking care of a seriously ill young nurse with a mysterious illness. A fellow intern, Dr. Rob Inman, and I were taking turns staying up every night for weeks with her trying both to diagnose and treat a condition that had caused her to have strange bleeding disorders, fevers, and repeated hemorrhages inside her brain. I had already spent almost six months on call every day and every other night in a rigorous training program in internal medicine, so my chronic fatigue went almost unnoticed. Several of my colleagues had mentioned that my eyes had a slight yellow cast and were continually bloodshot, but I attributed that to long sleepless nights on duty.

I also noticed that every morning after I showered and dried my hair with a blow-dryer sweat formed on my forehead, but I thought it was just a little too hot in my room and took no other step than to turn down the thermostat. I didn't notice then that the temperature in my apartment was already 62°. In fact I did nothing until a dull aching pain in the lower left side of my abdomen failed to go away.

While I was in the emergency department admitting a patient to the coronary care unit, I asked a surgical resident to examine my abdomen. He laughingly told me to hop up on the nearest table, but his face took on a strange look when he felt my belly. I had a massively enlarged spleen.

*He also said that I looked a little pale and felt hot. He took
my temperature; I had a temperature of 105°.*

*I checked my own blood count and realized that the res-
ident was right about my paleness. I was profoundly anemic, and more frighteningly my white blood cell count was
elevated. I made a blood smear to examine under the microscope as I had done on hundreds of patients before. I
saw a profusion of bizarre and strangely misshapen white
blood cells. I asked a lab technician to look at the smear
and tell me what she thought. She looked up from the microscope and with boredom asked, "How long has your patient had leukemia?" I told her it was my blood smear, and
she quickly said, averting her eyes, that it was probably just
mono. I had had infectious mononucleosis in college—and
you don't get it twice.*

*It all came together: the insidious onset of fever, anemia,
an enlarged spleen, jaundice probably representing liver involvement, and an increased number of abnormal-looking
white blood cells. I realized the most likely diagnosis was
acute lymphocytic leukemia—in someone my age, most likely
fatal.*

*I asked a faculty member in the medical school to be my
personal physician, and my apprehensions were multiplied
when he was concerned enough to suggest a bone marrow
examination. Leukemic cells are produced in the bone marrow, and taking a sample confirms the diagnosis of malignancy.*

*I knew the outcome of the disease even with radiation and
chemotherapy, and I didn't want either painful process and
wished the disease to take its natural course. Over the next
several weeks my temperature rose to a high of 106.3°, my
body ached in bone-wrenching pain, my eyes took on a permanent yellow tinge, and my gums bled. Numerous blood
samples were sent to the Centers for Disease Control (CDC)
and that blood-letting left me more anemic than I was when
my illness began.*

*I was too sick to work, too sick to eat, too sick to sleep.
I was no longer a doctor—I was a patient.*

*After about a month my illness remitted. Test results from the blood sent to the CDC showed that I had not been involved in a leukemic process but had in fact been infected by a virus, specifically cytomegalovirus. This is a viral infection that often produces a syndrome much like infectious mononucleosis and also has many symptoms in common with leukemia. The same tests on the blood of the young nurse I had stayed up so many nights taking care of confirmed she had cytomegalovirus, too. Like mononucleosis, it is a self-limited disease, and soon I was well and back to work again.*

*But I shall never forget what it was like to be "on the other side of the needle." To be a really good doctor, you have to be a patient at least once. Lessons we all learn, but the sooner the better.*

B. B. D.

# Lessons

## Steven E. Frank, M.D.

It began as a lump discovered late one night in a hasty-on-call shower. It was nestled up behind pectoralis major deep in my axilla. The lump was soft, not fixed, and nontender. Had it been a patient's axilla I probably would have said, "Lipoma—nothing to fret over," and told him to forget about it. But it was mine.

I asked an attending surgeon to have a look. "Lipoma," he said. "No sweat." But on examining me further he found a similar smaller mass contralaterally. Then he said: "Let's watch them for a while."

During the next few months, the lumps became more prominent. The one on the left enlarged, became softer, regressed, and enlarged again. The small one on the right became hard. The attending checked them a second and third time. He decided to remove them and told me to check in in three days.

I went to the program director to ask for a day or two off. He felt the lumps. "Any weight loss? Chest film lately? Fever?"

"No weight loss, normal chest film, no symptoms." It dawned on me: he was asking the lymphoma workup. "If that was my axilla, I'd want those things out pronto," he said and walked away.

The more I thought about it, the more scared I became: I was a 33-year-old man with a nonregressing firm rubbery mass, painless, waxing and waning, and a history of infectious mononucleosis. I even had pruritus. It all came together: Hodgkin's.

I was in-house on call all weekend and was becoming edgy. I had my preoperative CBC done and read the smear myself. It was totally normal, but that didn't help. I studied my medical texts, and by Monday morning I had a diagnosis: Hodgkin's disease, stage IA, maybe even IIA.

At noon I checked into the surgical department. "Hello, I'm Mary Jane," said a nurse I've known forever. "I'll be taking care of you today." She took a history, checked my vitals, and put me in a room.

"Take off *all* your clothes and put this on, open at the back," she said, handing me a gown.

"I'm not wearing a damned dress!"

"Yes you are."

"No I'm not . . ."

A few minutes later, properly gowned, I was brought a preop. Mary Jane bemoaned the fact that it was oral. It seemed she'd sold raffle tickets to the ER nurses to see who'd give me my shots. She also brought a shaving kit and instructed me to prep myself.

After a 2½-hour wait, I was in the OR, on the table, IV

in and running. We waited half an hour for the attending physician, who was in a meeting. We made small talk, but my eyes were fixed on a pair of blunt rakes on the Mayo. By the time the attending showed up I was fully convinced that ripping out the IV and dashing off down the hall would have been an excellent move.

I was later told I had "a little anxiety in there." Apparently, I hyperventilated, wouldn't lie down, and turned white as a sheet. Antegrade amnesia being what it is, I recalled none of it except a funny taste in my mouth and a nurse in postop telling me I was finished. Emergence from anesthesia is like trying to swim in a vat full of Jell-O. I struggled to stay awake. My eyes wouldn't focus. I became somehow convinced that if I fell asleep, I'd quit breathing.

The anesthesiologist came in. "Just lipomas," he said. "You're fine."

From there on it was no sweat. I dozed back off. An intern came in and wrote "Where's the beef?" on my belly. I was wheeled to my room and everybody had a party while I slept it off, or so I'm told.

I also learned some valuable lessons. All the people I'd seen that day I'd worked with on major cases. I had known their level of competence. Yet, even though it turned out that my surgery was so minor I probably could have done it myself, I had been terrified. I later thought of how it is with sick patients who must face surgery alone, among strangers whose competence and kindness have yet to be proved. I hope I never forget it.

# INSIDE THE DIAGNOSIS

## David M. Worthen, M.D.

The beginning was innocent. In July 1985 I received a shock from a hand-held electric drill. Within a week I'd recovered and felt fortunate to be alive.

But this minor accident heralded a permanent change in my life. I passed through the transparent curtain that separates physician from patient: I moved inside the diagnosis.

I have always enjoyed good health and was successful in competitive swimming and running. An ophthalmologist, I took pleasure in performing microsurgery. Approaching age 50 I feared any disability that would interfere with providing for my wife of 27 years and our five children. By the following November, however, progressive weakness of my left arm forced me to abandon performing any more surgery and prompted consultation at a university neurology department.

The differential diagnosis was broad; a major concern was a motor-neuron syndrome. I was relieved by the consultant's conclusion: the injury from the shock seemed isolated to my left arm, with some damage to the cord, causing long tract findings in my left leg. I was able to continue administration, education, and research.

During the summer my running times improved and I thought I was on the path to recovery.

Over Labor Day weekend I had a fever and headache. I tried to write a note to myself and found I couldn't use my

52

right hand. The fever spontaneously broke and I felt normal the next day, but within the next few weeks I had the onset of fasciculations in the fine muscles of my right hand, which progressed to my right forearm and shoulder. I also noticed spontaneous fasciculations in my left thigh. My strength was ebbing.

With my rapid decline in the fall of 1986, more associates and co-workers expressed concern and offered help. I still traveled frequently, but found it more difficult to haul luggage laden with papers and reports. I was amazed by the automatic, solicitous assistance from strangers with whom I was traveling. As my clumsiness increased, I turned to aides for help.

My mood swung from despair to euphoria, hope to loneliness; I saw dreams lost. The reality of death slithered into my consciousness like a serpent and punctured and numbed my waking hours.

On March 30, 1987, a second consultant confirmed the serpent's bite with an unequivocal diagnosis of amyotrophic lateral sclerosis (Lou Gehrig's disease). Suddenly I was one of those ''other people'' to whom I thought these things always happen. The consultant wondered if the ALS might have been precipitated by the trauma of the electric shock. To me, it didn't matter; the reality and the consequences were the same. The death sentence had been declared and the prison of my body defined.

Noble Lou Gehrig's—it causes progressive loss of most voluntary movement over a two- to three-year period, eventually robbing its victim of speech, swallowing, and respiration, but leaving his mind alert and all his senses intact. Unlike Alzheimer's disease, severe trauma, or cancer, ALS does not destroy the intellect or disfigure the body. Unlike AIDS, it does not endanger a spouse or family—like AIDS, it is a demanding test of their devotion.

When the diagnosis was made I felt transformed. Suddenly, the physician's desire to heal was transformed into a patient's desire for help, cure into caring, certainty into hope. Throughout my years of teaching, I had tried to impress students and residents with the importance of crawling inside the patient and trying to experience what the physician's words meant to him. I recalled the many, many patients referred to me with "hopeless" conditions. I remembered how so many were relieved when I chose words other than "disease," or "cancer," or "blindness." Above all, I stressed to my students the need to leave every patient with hope. Hope makes the horizon bright, the pain less, and each day worth living. I often tried to discern what patients wanted to hear, what they could accept, what was better told only to a loved one. I now found myself in that position, wanting to hear the truth, willing and able to accept anything, wanting to share the reality with the persons I loved as the kindest framework within which to cope.

"Are you sure?" "Could they be wrong?" "What can I do?" asked friends and colleagues. I listened to their accounts of pain and the torment of their (or their loved one's) own illnesses. Many wondered about the impact of my illness on them. And their emotions shone on their faces. I saw denial, anger, sorrow, disbelief, revulsion, recognition, sympathy, empathy, as each relived the secret terror of death and dying.

From here, from inside the diagnosis, I am impressed with the universal need that all people have to care and to give support in so many ways. Yet most leave room for the individual to assert his independence as best he can. Every day there is a new loss, every day a new insight, every day a new frontier. Every day I realize that joy comes not only from giving help, but from accepting help.

I draw strength from a lifetime filled with achievement, optimism, and curiosity. I see progressive handicap as a challenge and an opportunity to strive in a way that the able-bodied seldom experience. I use my ingenuity to discover new ways of accomplishing activities as my bodily functions deteriorate. I vow denial to the strength-sapping saprophytes of depression, despair, frustration, and fear.

As the patient, I find that the second-to-second hurt of living the diagnosis contrasts with the episodic pain of the physician's declaring a diagnosis, then walking away. As a physician, I have come full cycle: I live both sides of the diagnosis.

I realized an inner peace when my sentence had been declared, my time defined, my remaining tasks listed. To know the time of death and to be able to share with the people I love the emotions denied to those who depart so rapidly is a gift that compensates for the slow dissolution of movement. As physical ability is lost, there is no lessening of my will to bump against whatever obstacles I meet and to achieve whatever I can achieve.

Dr. Worthen passed away April 14, 1988.

# A Sensitive Subject

## Elliott B. Oppenheim, M.D.

When my medical school class began there were 64 eager students, and 64 students eventually finished four years later. I recall each year the story surrounding the one who did not make it and was replaced.

From the first day we were told how small our class size was; it was obvious to anyone who had come from the larger universities. One Berkeley graduate said, "I had more people than this in my organic lab!"

The newness of the school soon faded, but the excitement of histology, physiology, and courses I can no longer remember propelled us through the first quarter.

Tight groups of friends readily developed, but one person

seemed to remain anonymous even within this small group of 64. It was the classics major, dark-haired, with round-rimmed tortoise-shell glasses, soft-spoken, who, when we were in social groups, was always alone. He did not play touch football, throw the Frisbee, or enter political discussions about the Vietnam situation.

As students we were thinking axons, glutamine transferase, and polysaccharides, but he was still marveling over Virgil, Cicero, and Chaucer. His father had wanted him to be a physician, and Ted took the requisite premedical courses, applied to medical school, and was accepted. Shortly after class began, he found his enthusiasm was simply not in pancreatic acini, loops of Henle, or intestinal villi. How could he ever hold his father's admiration if he left medical school?

He and I discussed this predicament one day at lunch. It was late in the southern California fall, just before finals, when we lunched and shared secrets. I told him about my desire to become a novelist and he related his wish to translate Greek classics. He did not want to be a physician.

Like a small boat at sea tossed in a storm, the class was overwhelmed by finals. After Christmas break, there we were, back again. This time it was anatomy, more histology, and physiology. I seem to remember we were learning about red blood cells in afternoon lab when our class president entered the room.

"Ted committed suicide last night. He overdosed on barbs," he said. "The parents want no remembrances."

We were shocked, but little was ever said. Few of us realized the loss. No one had known him! The administration made no effort to give us any understanding of the complex issues, and I don't think that the department of psychiatry even knew about it until years later. Classes went on without an ectopic beat, much less a run of ventricular tachycardia.

A student replaced Ted within a week and ultimately did well. He wanted to be a physician.

Despite our small class size and a number of small

groups, Ted had remained a distant outsider. He was in every way unaffiliated and anonymous. He had a girl friend, but she was 300 miles away. His parents, with whom he had been both distant and close, made their goals and his need to achieve them a clear contingency.

The rugged medical students were concerned with new anatomy vocabulary and excluded their paternal role with a classmate. It was not an optimal time for class support since we, too, were new. *We* barely knew one another.

So there he was without an acceptable solution . . . except one.

The first days of medical school are like an angel food cake in the making. There is stress in the transition from lay person to medical student, and if a door is slammed prematurely, the cake can fall.

A small class does not guarantee closeness, but support systems do guarantee, at least, the probable identification of those of us with serious emotional problems. In our second year one professor invited small discussion sessions to his home. These groups of 12 ostensibly dealt with ethical issues in medicine, but the topics were far-ranging and allowed us an opportunity to interact.

The troubled student is usually identifiable if one looks carefully. Like rales in pneumonia, loneliness, anxiety, and drug use (including alcohol) are important signs in the presuicide.

I believe that medical schools should conduct "get-acquainted" groups led by faculty members with eight to 12 students meeting every four weeks. Most physicians who would volunteer to host such a group would be sensitive enough to spot a troubled student. The faculty person would also be seen as approachable in a time of need.

While it may be impossible to rework a medical student's life even with empathetic friends, for many, medical school is the beginning of psychotherapy or psychoanalysis that eventually does create a happier physician.

Physicians are fearful about approaching patients as people and worry, "If the patient has the same problem I do, how can I help if I have not helped myself?'' We have an aversion to emotional turmoil as medical students that persists in the physician. But as we learn to approach our patients, we must also learn to approach our colleagues.

Parents wish success for their offspring, but it is the child who must be successful. Vicarious parental success is an inordinate and unfair burden for a medical student.

Faculty meetings and administrative sensitivity are important adjuncts to prevention of suicide in medical students, but as in many medical issues, the answer literally lies in our hands. We must knock on a door every once in a while, risk being intrusive, and learn to talk with our brethren about a sensitive subject.

No other profession has anything remotely resembling what is called an internship. After four years of a medical education and a diploma, a young person with an M.D. degree is still not really a doctor until he or she has been through an internship. In fact, doctors cannot be licensed to practice medicine until they have served a year in that grueling enterprise.

During an internship, young men and women are asked to take on the responsibility of life and death, are pushed to the limits of physical and emotional endurance, and are watched constantly for the first sign of error; it is the crucible in which all physicians are created. It is the most hated and the most loved year in any doctor's life.

In the past, many programs prohibited interns even from being married. They were made to live in the hospital (interns and residents still bear the name "house staff"), and many interns were required to work every day and every other night. Nowadays the entire internship and residency process is under reform because of the realization that the physical and mental stress of the internship are not good for the trainees or their patients, but it is still the proving ground for any doctor.

My own internship at Vanderbilt Medical Center in Nashville, Tennessee, was an every-other-night program. Interns worked seven days a week without letup. A typical day would begin at 6 AM and end the next evening at 6 PM; a seriously ill patient might keep you up even longer. If you were lucky you went home for dinner, but you usually found yourself too tired to eat, collapsing asleep on the couch with your clothes on. The alarm clock woke you at 5 in the morning, time to start another 36 straight hours. Some professors

59

*deadpanned that the only thing wrong with an every-other-night program was that you missed seeing half the cases.*

*Of course, the intent of the grueling pace is to see everything, to confront as many challenging cases as possible in a year in order to prepare yourself for the unexpected medical world. With the traineeship comes a nametag that says M.D., affixed to a new, starched, white uniform.*

*A search of that uniform would reveal the following—a stethoscope, a battery-operated paging device, a reflex hammer, tongue depressors, an assortment of vials and test tubes, penlights, safety pins for testing sensation to touch, rubber tubing used for tourniquets in blood drawing, a tape measure, a combination otoscope/ophthalmoscope for examining the ears and eyes, lab slips, cotton swabs, syringes, needles, ampules of emergency medicines, glass microscope slides, index cards imprinted with patients' names and clinical histories, and, most important, what interns call their* peripheral brain, *a pocket-sized but thick notebook stuffed with every known medical fact, emergency procedure, and phone number interns think they will ever need.*

*You'll find interns in teaching hospitals working up* new *patients, performing lumbar punctures and bone marrow exams, running to the lab, inserting bladder catheters, going to lectures, looking at x-rays, running to the ER, presenting cases on rounds, lancing boils, running to cardiac arrests, examining all sorts of things under a microscope, teaching third-year medical students, doing CPR, sewing up wounds, running to the telephone, reading the latest medical journals, removing lice, changing IVs, wheeling patients down the hall, running to the ICU, taking ECGs, drawing their own blood to transfuse premature infants, grabbing some food from a tray, all the while trying to comfort the sick and console grief-stricken families.*

*Strangely, none of this apparently frightens off interns, but what they live in fear of is their first real assignment. And, God forbid, what if it's to be the only doctor in the emergency room!*

B. B. D.

# Internship—July 1962

## Leonard G. Dauber, M.D.

He was nervous and he knew it. He had slept fitfully the night before, anticipating the alarm set to wake him at 6:30 A.M. He washed and shaved, then dressed in his uniform whites. He bolted down his morning coffee, a quick cup of instant made without thinking. His thoughts were elsewhere. He remembered to put his stethoscope into his right side jacket pocket, his pen and pencil into the upper left pocket, and his notebook and percussion hammer into his lower left pocket. A safety pin was attached through the first buttonhole of his jacket and he knotted a length of soft rubber tubing through a belt loop.

Today he was starting his postgraduate apprenticeship. He was an intern and was to begin his rotation in the emergency room.

He was early: the clock on the emergency room wall said 7:45 AM. No matter. He knew the tightness in his abdomen would not go away until he became involved in his work. The emergency area was quiet. In the cubicles, crisp white sheets covered the high-wheeled gurneys that were his examining tables. All of the booths were empty; the curtains were pulled back in anticipation of patients to be examined.

He walked to the nursing station to check in. His instructions had been to relieve the intern on duty and take over. He knew this meant that he had to complete the ex-

amination of patients held in the emergency room over-
night and make a judgment to dismiss them or admit them
to the hospital ward. He knew he would also be responsible for all new patients after eight o'clock. He looked at
his watch. In ten minutes he would begin his internship:
5½ days a week plus every other night and every other
weekend.

The nurse at the station was clearing her desk of paper.
"Miss Sullivan, R.N.," her nametag read. She half looked
at him as he introduced himself and began to explain that
this was his first day. "Joe, he's the intern on last night, is
sleeping. Why'n'cha go have a cup of coffee and I'll call
you when it gets busy." "But," he began to protest. "Go
on with you now," she said, just a bit of Irish brogue creep-
ing into her speech.

The hospital coffee was no better than the cup of instant
he had had an hour or so before, but he sipped it slowly.
He was eager to get back to the "Pit," as he had learned
the emergency room was called irreverently, but reluctant
to face the nurse without complying with her instructions.

After half an hour, his impatience to be doing something,
anything, pushed him back to the emergency room. Miss
Sullivan was there to welcome him again. "Where've you
been?" she asked with a smile. "There's a patient in the
booth there for you." She pointed to a cubicle, its curtains
drawn, and handed him the standard emergency room sheet.
The patient was a 17-year-old boy who had abdominal pain;
the log-in time had been 8:13 AM.

He turned and walked toward the cubicle, with the differential diagnosis of abdominal pain whirling through his
mind. The anxiety he had awoken with that morning, and
had been trying to contain, heightened. This was his first
patient as an intern.

He parted the curtains and reached for his stethoscope
for what comfort the cold metal and plastic tubing could
provide. "Good morning," he began, striving for that tone
of brisk efficiency and competence he had admired in his
professors. He took the patient's history; abdominal pain

was sharp, beginning at the umbilicus the evening before, then gradually intensifying and moving into the right lower part of the abdomen, where the pain was now localized; slight fever, but no vomiting, diarrhea, or bowel movements. He was comfortable with knees drawn up but less so in any other position. He had never been sick before. "Well, it could be just about anything," he thought; all of the possibilities were still fluttering about in his mind.

He had the patient undress and put on a clean examining gown. He checked the fact sheet and found that his nurse had recorded vital signs, all normal except temperature, which was 38.0°C. He started his examination just as he had been taught in medical school, grateful to be caught up in the methodical approach of beginning at the head and working down. He found no abnormalities until he came to the abdominal examination. The patient's abdomen was markedly tender, particularly in the right lower quadrant. The tenderness was referred to the right lower quadrant of the abdomen on further examination elsewhere in the abdomen, and the muscles over the right side of the abdomen were tense and did not yield to inward pressure. A smile began to form on his face as he worked. A lecture on the acute abdomen from his surgical clerkship in medical school snapped into memory. He remembered. "McBurney," he murmured several times. He straightened up, put an examining sheet over the patient, and instructed him to stay on the gurney. He left the booth, closing the curtains, and walked with a jaunty, almost cocky swagger back to the nursing station. He felt secure in his judgment, and the anxiety of the minutes before seemed in the distant past. It had taken him no more than ten minutes. He had made his first diagnosis by himself and he was elated and gratified, confident and proud at penetrating the difficulties of the patient's presentation with such celerity.

"Miss Sullivan," he began, "please call the surgical resident. I believe that boy has acute appendicitis. He has signs all localized to McBurney's point in the right abdomen. I want a complete blood count and then we'll have the surgeons see him.''

Miss Sullivan smiled again. "I've already drawn his blood, Doctor, and the surgical resident was called 20 minutes ago and should be here shortly. I've called the surgical ward and they are expecting the patient just as soon as you've finished examining him.''

His internship had begun.


# THIS IS MY BLOOD

## Joseph B. Vander Veer, Jr., M.D.


"The Professor will see you now, Miss." The secretary replaced the handset as the third-year medical student rose and headed toward the office of the Professor of Hematology.

"How nice to see you." The Professor motioned her to be seated. "What's on your mind?"

"It's no one particular thing, Professor. Actually, I'm a little embarrassed to be here, since it isn't any earthshaking matter, really." She avoided his eyes and looked down at the carpet. Her blouse was slightly faded; one of the collar tabs was outside the lapel of the short white jacket she was wearing, the cuffs of which were frayed. The nametag, he recognized, was just like the one he had worn as a student—simple first and last names. No Dr. or M.D. such as the interns and residents could wear. "I guess I'm just discouraged."

The Professor asked about things at home, thinking he

might turn up something. He knew she had received scholarship funds (he was on the selection committee), and she had a part-time job on Saturdays in the coagulation research lab, which he headed. As he listened, he realized the problem was not social or financial.

"It seems like what we're doing is a lot of drill," continued the student. "I know the workups are important, but sometimes they seem so useless, take so long, and hardly any of the profs read them."

He realized she was being frank. He harked back to his own clinical clerkship. How little had changed. Despite computers, fancy scanners, and new miracle drugs, teaching and learning bedside medicine were much the same: one student with one patient critiqued by one professor. He, too, had complained that his workups were never read. It was the intern's dictated workup that ended up on the chart, the official document, so to speak. And although the lowly clerks were able to write orders for treatments and medications, they could not be carried out. Even in the student's fourth year, given status by the name "externship," he had to have all his orders countersigned by the resident before the nurses would honor them. No, the drill hadn't changed.

He swiveled around in the chair to look across the campus. "During my training, we had some of the same discouragements. I remember one student on the hematology wards who voiced the same problems, doing lots of work with little feedback, having some knowledge but not enough to be trusted with the management of a case, looking like a doctor in dress and manner, considered by patients and families to *be* one, but frustrated and helpless nonetheless."

"That's it exactly," she said. The Professor, who had continued to look out the window as he spoke, now turned back.

"This student had a night job in the blood bank, on all night once a week. He was responsible for setting up the presurgical blood for the next day and for responding to any emergency that arose. Back then, we didn't have any component therapy, so when someone was bleeding rapidly you had to give fresh blood.

"We had a procedure called walk-in donors, calling in folks whose blood type was known, when fresh blood was needed. You had to call up the donor, have him come in, draw his blood, refrigerate it while you did a crossmatch, which took an hour. If it was OK, then you'd release the blood. Some of the labile clotting factors—the ones we quick-freeze nowadays—and the platelets would drop off pretty fast. I'm not sure how effective it really was.

"The clerk on our service had worked up a 17-year-old girl with drug-induced thrombocytopenia; she came in covered with purpuric blotches."

The student had seen one patient like that already, skin mottled by hemorrhages because of the low platelet count. She remembered reading about the disease.

"About three days after admission, this girl began to hemorrhage. It happened about 7 o'clock, after the medical students had gone home, on the evening nursing shift. Her blood pressure dropped and she passed out—I think it was in the bathroom, where her mother found her during visiting hours—and the resident sent off some specimens stat to request walk-in donors, since the platelets from fresh blood were the only thing that could save her.

"The clerk happened to be on duty in the blood bank that night and recognized her name on the requisition. When he typed her, he found that she was the same type that he was. So, he drew a specimen of his own blood and crossmatched it against hers. It matched. I remember his saying how hard it was to jam that big needle into his own antecubital vein! You can imagine the rest."

"Did she stop bleeding?" the student asked as she sat forward on her chair.

"The clerk said he got a bit woozy because he drew off two pints. He took them up to the ward himself, properly and anonymously numbered, of course. The charge nurse didn't know him because she worked evenings, but the girl's mother saw him at the desk and called out to him, brought him down to the room because her daughter had been asking for him—seems she considered him to be her doctor over all the other house staff and attendings. He went down and sat by her, taking her pulse, noting her cool, moist hands and pallor, watching as the nurse and intern on call checked the numbers against the slips, then hung up the bottles of blood. Then he was paged and had to go.

"She did stop—the clerk knew because he didn't get any more requests for blood for her that night, and in the morning she looked vastly different when he returned in the grand rounds entourage. Despite his excitement, he told no one but me, and I guess he told me because he fell asleep on rounds and I poked him to stay awake." The Professor rose to come around to the student's side. "She recovered her platelets and was discharged a few days later. Sometimes we need to be reminded that students do make a difference."

The student seemed more erect, he thought, as he escorted her out. He closed the door behind her, sat on the edge of the desk, and gazed across the campus, across the years, wondering how much that delicate young patient, and his moonlighting blood bank job, had influenced his decision to become a hematologist.


# TEACHINGS OF THE HEART

## Malinda H. Bell

"Who wants to sew a head laceration?" the emergency department resident asked. I glanced up from the chart I was completing, and he tossed me the runner: ''52-year-old white male with head laceration. No loss of consciousness. Alcohol on breath.'' Same old stuff, I thought.

I was at the end of my emergency department clerkship, and much of what I did as a senior student was by reflex. I grabbed the laceration tray, size 6 gloves, and 5-0 nylon suture. I could smell the alcohol through the curtain, so I wasn't surprised to find my patient passed out on the cart. I woke him and gave the required spiel about the procedure, risks, and aftercare. The resident had already taken the history and completed the physical, leaving me to practice my suturing and allowing him to return to the controlled chaos of the night shift.

I adjusted the light to shine directly on the oozing cut and decided as I sat down that 30 minutes of sewing might be a nice respite. I deadened the edges of the cut, marveling that the patient didn't flinch as I pricked his scalp a dozen times.

Reflecting on the gruesome sight of a patient passed out on the gurney, hair matted with blood, I was amazed at how my attitude had changed in the last four years. In my first months as a medical student, I was called a ''softie'' when I cried about patients; being a woman only made it worse. Classmates and physicians told me, ''You get too emotionally involved with patients. You will never be a 'good' doctor.'' Now, as I neared the end of medical school and thought about my composure tonight, I supposed the transformation from ''softie'' to ''good doctor'' had occurred. After all, wasn't I treating this patient and yet ''removing myself'' from his condition? When had the magic moment dawned, and why didn't bells ring and drums roll? I felt pretty smug.

Suddenly the curtain around my cubicle flew open and the resident shouted, ''We need you in the trauma room!'' I glanced at the snoring mass under the sterile blue towels and knew he wouldn't mind the interruption.

I nearly ran into a young man cradling an elderly man in his arms. The youth was sobbing, ''It's his heart . . . my daddy's gonna die.'' We rushed the father to the trauma room, and I gasped. His face was a splotchy bluish-purple, and he wasn't moving. "Dusky" had been a textbook term until that moment. I had never seen it before, and now I would never forget it.

The staff went about their duties carefully, deliberately, and quickly. I scrunched against the wall, not knowing quite how to help. A doctor looked directly at me and commanded: "YOU, continue cardiac resuscitation." I wobbled to the patient's side, feeling very unsure of myself. I measured three finger-widths above the xiphoid, carefully positioned my hands, and made the first compression. The feel of warm flesh and hard ribs giving way beneath my hands was startling. IV lines were placed, blood gases drawn, heart tracing done, and drugs infused appropriately.

Suddenly, the patient's face turned red. He fought the endotracheal tube for a few seconds, but soon quit struggling—and then, we lost him. We worked until the sweat dripped from my forehead to my hands and then between my fingers to his chest. Defibrillation, drugs—nothing rekindled his tired heart.

The doctor in charge terminated the code, and we stood in respectful silence. I stared at the still chest and recalled the waiting son. He had given his father to us with hope. It seemed wrong to me that strangers should be the witnesses of death, perhaps the most intimate moment in a life. I felt indebted to this stranger; I was indeed a "softie" and to be anything else was unpardonable.

I stayed by the patient's side and stared at the imprint of my hands on his chest. "I'm sorry," I whispered. A resident who overhead me and also noticed the marks said, "Don't worry, kid. They will disappear before the body's cold."

Knowing he did not understand me and not wanting to explain, I mumbled, "Thanks." As I left to return to the clamor down the hall, I knew my marks on that man's body were transient, but his mark on me would last a lifetime.

# MRS. STRAUSS AND MABEL

## Adria Burrows

The other day I admitted Mable Fairfax, a 75-year-old woman with organic brain syndrome. She was a thin woman with sunken eyes and gray, wavy hair. Mabel didn't know where she was or even if she had a daughter, and as I examined her, she kept asking, "Are you a doctor? Are you a doctor?" She sat in her wheelchair with a towel around her shoulders for a shawl. Her crooked fingers frequently stroked her chin. She seemed content in her new surroundings and sat quietly.

Mrs. Strauss, the other patient in the room, was a short woman, also in her 70s, who was plump and had a mean disposition. She loved to turn her radio on loudly to annoy the nurses, and once she threw food at the blood drawer. All you had to do was walk into her room and she would greet you with "What are you doing here? Get out and leave me alone." Otherwise, she would sit by the window, quietly peeling oranges that she liked to throw at people who bothered her.

To my surprise, Mrs. Strauss took a liking to Mabel. As soon as Mabel was wheeled into the room, Mrs. Strauss got up and said to the nurse, "Be careful, won't you? You'll bang her chair against the bed. What kind of a nurse are you?" Two of the nurses lifted Mabel into her bed as Mrs. Strauss supervised with comments like "What're you doing? Be more careful. You people don't know anything."

She stood and watched them carefully as they tucked Mabel into the bed, and after they left, she smoothed the blankets over Mabel's frail body.

"Are you a doctor?" Mabel asked Mrs. Strauss.

"No," came the answer. Mabel closed her eyes and leaned back in bed, exhausted from nothing. Mrs. Strauss stood next to her and began to comb Mabel's hair in silence.

Mrs. Strauss seemed to consider herself Mabel's guardian. She fed her, saving anything she didn't eat for later, washed her hands and face with a wet washcloth each morning, and chased the nurses out of the room when they came to take Mabel's temperature. The radio never played loudly and the oranges lay unpeeled in a basket.

Mabel barely knew what was going on but smiled when her face was wiped and fell to sleep peacefully as Mrs. Strauss hummed to her. She couldn't remember Mrs. Strauss' name, although she was told what it was over and over again.

The day Mabel had to leave the hospital, Mrs. Strauss helped her into the wheelchair, straightened a blanket on her lap, and kissed her good-bye on the cheek. Mrs. Strauss watched as Mabel was wheeled out of the room and then sat down by the window. Her fingers toyed with a string on her housecoat as she gazed at Mabel's empty bed.

"Are you all right?" I asked her.

"Some people just can't take care of themselves. You know, Mabel needed me. I haven't felt needed for years, Doctor." Her voice was soft and her head tilted to the side.

Suddenly, as if she had woken from a trance, she walked to the radio and turned up the volume. "Now let me alone!" she yelled. "Can't you see I want to be by myself?" As I left the room, I was just able to catch a glimpse of Mabel being wheeled around the corner down the hall.

# LIES AND RUDE FOOLS

## Robert G. Westphal, M.D.

Children are an incredible race, resilient yet sensitive beyond our own capacity to believe. They have not yet learned to be fools, they are purely simple; they have not yet learned to be rude, they are only honest. But they know the importance of a lie.

My patient had two sons, ages 10 and 12, and they had not been to visit their father in the hospital since his urgent, middle-of-the-night admission three days before. The grandparents and my patient's new wife (who was not the boys' mother) were upset by their own grief and uncertain whether the effect of seeing their dying father in such a severe state of illness and confusion would be harmful to the children. I suggested that a brief dose of reality would be much better than the many fantasies and imagined horrors that might be in their young minds.

It required a trip of some distance, but the visit was duly made. We went up together after a few brief words of explanation. Dad was febrile and sweating; his skin was very yellow; his abdomen was very swollen. His respirations were grunting, his breath short, his words only occasionally intelligible.

He tried to speak to me, or to the children, I couldn't be sure. There was an awkward silence; there were big eyes and, I confess, some moist ones. The youngest, and shortest, blurted out that he had gotten a B+ in social studies.

The oldest echoed with regard to math. Dad, who is my age, struggled and groped to communicate and finally mumbled, ''That's great!'' More silence, but less awkward.

And then a small hand, and then two, reached out and touched and stroked their father's arm. ''You're going to be all right, Dad, you really are.'' Such a lie, which one shares, is sometimes not a lie at all, but a great and ennobling verity without which we would all recognize this sad madness for what it may be.

Later, I had to respond to the inquiries about the ''tubes'' in the arm and the oxygen and other physical signs and concerns. But the bravest moment had already happened. It took place before we went up to visit. I had offered some rudimentary explanations and then asked my attentive young audience if there were any questions. ''Yeah, I got just one: is he going to make it?''

I, too, know the importance of a lie and when to use it. This was not such a time, for I knew I was not dealing with the rude fools we adults are. Our children may be the only honest people left.


# The Surprise Party

## Harold I. Eist, M.D.

In understanding the experience of mentally ill individuals, we should recognize the courage they often exhibit even while engaging in superficial ordinary human interactions. Unless we appreciate this, their responses of isolation and withdrawal because of interpersonal terror will seem inexplicable. Two clinical examples help to clarify this point.

An alcoholic woman began talking about her son, who had been psychotic since childhood, and I wondered if there would ever be any end to her grief. Alcohol had destroyed her liver, but it had not washed away the grief. She mentioned with a slight smile that finally she was beginning to accept the many losses her son's illness represented.

"We had him home from the hospital Sunday, and Mary, the friend I told you about who also has a schizophrenic son, brought him over. The two boys have known each other since they were kids and there they were, both of them on the couch, acting like the other one didn't exist."

Her remark took me back 17 years to a medication group I had run for chronically schizophrenically ill patients at a Veterans Administration hospital. During my weekly sessions with the group, as each of the ten assiduously avoided eye contact with the others, I often thought, "You guys don't need a psychiatrist—you need an air traffic control operator."

Six weeks prior to my leaving this group, I announced I was moving on to another service. Each patient responded by firmly fixing his eyes on a distant point. I wondered if there was any concern on the part of the group members at my leaving, but I couldn't tell for sure.

As the group assembled at the last meeting, one of the members, who was uncharacteristically well groomed, emptied a bag of doughnuts in the center of the group-room table. Each member of the group filed to the table and took a doughnut.

"The last one's for you, Doc," one of them said. "It's a surprise party." Suddenly it hit me that these terribly isolated men had gotten together in spite of their fearfulness and had planned a party for me. Furthermore, in the face of crippling illness, they had carried it off.

We ate our doughnuts silently, no one looking at anyone else, and then we discussed medications. I shook hands with each of them, and someone said, "Hope you enjoy your new job."

"Me too," I answered, full of sadness, gratitude, and new-found understanding.

# THE GOAL

## Jane Doe

I am the wife of a sixth-year surgical resident. My husband is in a highly selective surgical subspecialty. In a field replete with top-notch members, my husband competes and succeeds. The price of his success has been the loss of a meaningful life outside the hospital milieu. The life-and-death events that my husband handles on a daily basis with skill, dedication, and empathy perhaps have served as catalysts in his change from a loving, caring husband and father to an exhausted, passive "boarder" who only occasionally arrives home during daylight hours.

The intensity of a surgeon's training has been tradition-bound to "break the man but not his mind." Eight years ago, when we married, my husband was a medical student. I listened to him, as class president, deliver his medical school's graduation speech, and I did so with a commitment to help him become the physician he dreamed of becoming—a healer, a surgeon ("The Goal"). As president of his medical school class, as a community leader in fund-raising, and as a Big Brother volunteer, my husband remained true to himself—a person whose humanistic ideals were embodied in the way he conducted his daily life.

During the first years of his surgery training, when I was teaching emotionally disturbed children and raising our daughter, I coped, only occasionally losing sight of The Goal. Coping involved emergency room visits to local hospitals when our daughter became ill (always, it seemed, at 3 AM on daddy's "on-call" nights), and one Christmas Eve ER trip that I still remember vividly. The miscarriage I was having was cleaned up without more than a small dose of Demerol and some handholding from a young nurse while my obstetrician complained that it would take too long for an anesthesiologist to arrive on this holiday night (and he wanted to get home). My husband was on call for surgery, and in his kindness as senior resident on duty, dismissed the other resident and intern, since it was a quiet night. This professional benevolence on his part and the lack of adequate staff backup left me alone that night. Although I recall having felt somewhat triumphant in knowing I could now cope with *anything* myself—even losing a child—The Goal suddenly seemed less important, as the emotional needs of our family continued to be neglected.

We endured as best we could. He, consumed in patient care and research (one of the more published residents at the medical center), while I taught school and taught his little girl to admire her daddy and understand that his growing absence was necessary to help other children who were less fortunate. And she endured. A little 4-year-old who was known by the hospital switchboard operators on a first-name basis. A 4-year-old who dreamed of becoming a nurse, in hopes of seeing her daddy more. A child who loved the precious few hours every other Sunday with her daddy, hours often spent taking off his 3-day-old socks and placing pillows under his head while Mommy tried to feed him in bed because he was too exhausted to sit at the kitchen table.

My husband will complete his residency in June—11 years of training counting medical school. He will, I am certain, make great strides in his field. Perhaps he will remember a few of the things his family endured for his chosen professional goal. The attorney who is handling the separation informs me that starting salaries are quite high in my husband's subspecialty. I remember the loans I gladly signed during the years of training to supplement his income, to pay the rent. Child support is assured to be more than adequate, the attorney says, but because I am now in law school, my future earnings will preclude "rehabilitative" maintenance. My "rehabilitation" will involve a mending of my heart, I tell this attorney.

We made it through medical school and most of residency. We coped for a long time, in our different ways. His patients should be grateful. Their bright young surgeon has been skillfully trained but selfishly possessed by a system that forgets that behind many good residents are their families, waiting.

# AGING AND CARING

## Paul E. Ruskin, M.D.

I was invited to present a lecture to a class of graduate nurses who were studying the "Psychosocial Aspects of Aging." I started my lecture with the following case presentation:

The patient is a white female who appears her reported age. She neither speaks nor comprehends the spoken word. Sometimes she babbles incoherently for hours on end. She is disoriented about person, place, and time. She does, however, seem to recognize her own name. I have worked with her for the past six months, but she still does not recognize me.

She shows complete disregard for her physical appearance and makes no effort whatsoever to assist in her own care. She must be fed, bathed, and clothed by others. Because she is edentulous, her food must be puréed, and because she is incontinent of both urine and stool, she must be changed and bathed often. Her shirt is generally soiled from almost incessant drooling. She does not walk. Her sleep pattern is erratic. Often she awakens in the middle of the night, and her screaming awakens others.

Most of the time she is very friendly and happy. However, several times a day she gets quite agitated without apparent cause. Then she screams loudly until someone comes to comfort her.

After the case presentation, I asked the nurses how they would feel about taking care of a patient such as the one described. They used words such as "frustrated," "hopeless," "depressed," and "annoyed" to describe how they would feel.

When I stated that I enjoyed taking care of her and that I thought they would, too, the class looked at me in disbelief. I then passed around a picture of the patient: my 6-month-old daughter.

After the laughter had subsided, I asked why it was so much more difficult to care for a 90-year-old than a 6-month-old with identical symptoms. We all agreed that it is physically easier to take care of a helpless baby weighing 15 pounds than a helpless adult weighing 100, but the answer seemed to go deeper than this.

The infant, we all agreed, represents new life, hope, and almost infinite potential. The demented senior citizen, on the other hand, represents the end of life, with little potential for growth.

We need to change our perspective. The aged patient is just as lovable as the child. Those who are ending their lives in the helplessness of old age deserve the same care and attention as those who are beginning their lives in the helplessness of infancy.

# FIVE PERFECT FINGERS

## John H. Vassall II, M.D.

I was a third-year medical student on the obstetrics service. I had already delivered more than three dozen babies, all warm, wiggling, light, and joyous little things that brought smiles to everyone's lips. Three dozen times I saw the tension and pain of childbirth turn instantly to pleasure with the newborn's first cry. How different it had been tonight!

I had just delivered the stillborn fetus of a diabetic primigravida. The mother was very obese and her diabetes had been out of control during her pregnancy. I had waited in agonizing silence for this baby. The collapsed skull entered the birth canal before complete cervical dilation had occurred. I spent an eternity whispering reassurances to the mother while waiting for passage of the baby's shoulders. Finally with a rush of fluid, the baby dropped, limp and heavy, into my hands like a bag of sand. I will never forget the awful weight of that baby. I cut the cord and quickly had the fetus removed from the room. When the placenta was delivered and my job done, I retreated to the call room, where I sat in heavy silence until I felt the obstetric resident's hand on my shoulder.

"It's time to show her the baby," he said. The image of what I had just seen was anything but pleasant.

"Hasn't she been through enough already?" I asked.

"She has to see the baby. Otherwise she'll never know."

The resident had already shown the fetus to the father,

who was now ready to give support to his wife. We surrounded the small cot where the baby's body lay, and the resident drew back the sheet. The mother began to cry.

"I want you to look closely at this baby," the resident said. "He has five perfect fingers on each hand. His arms and legs are perfectly developed and normal. His body is normal. Although the bones in the skull have shifted in the birth process, the head is nonetheless normally developed in every way."

We looked again at the small form on the cot; the tiny fingernails, the eyelashes, the little nose and ears, all perfectly formed and beautiful.

"You can have a normal baby," the resident said.

The resident and I left them alone with their baby. When I glanced back over my shoulder, the mother was still sobbing, but she was touching the tiny hand. I had had my first lesson in the art of medicine.

# SECOND OPINION

## Joseph E. Hardison, M.D.

Twenty years ago I was a medical resident. I remember one night I had seen three patients and none could be called interesting. Mr. Thomas was my fourth patient. His chief complaint was weakness. He had little spontaneity, his face was expressionless, his eyelids drooped, and his voice was nasal. My fatigue began to give way to excitement. Mr. Thomas was a very interesting patient. He answered yes to: Do you ever see double? Do you tire easily? Do you have trouble swallowing? Does food or water come back through your nose? Has your voice changed? Do your eyelids droop? Mr. Thomas wasn't impressed with the astuteness of my questions. If anything he became more apathetic. I had to strain to hear and understand him "Mr. Thomas, I think I know what is wrong with you. I want to give you a small dose of medicine in the vein of your arm." The response to edrophonium chloride was dramatic. His eyelids flew up, he sat upright, his face was mobile, and his voice resonant. I could hardly contain myself. I had heard and read about myasthenia gravis, and I had diagnosed my first case all by myself. "What do you think I have?" he asked. "Mr. Thomas, I believe you have a disease called myasthenia gravis. We will be able to help you." Something was wrong. The news seemed to sadden Mr. Thomas. He asked no questions about the disease or the treatment. The edrophonium chloride began to wear off; his eyelids drooped and his voice weakened. "Are you sure?" he nasalized. "I am almost positive," I replied, somewhat confused. Mr. Thomas told me he knew he had myasthenia gravis. I was put out. "Why didn't you tell me? Why did you let me go through the history and give you Tensilon when you knew all the time what was wrong with you?" "I am sorry," he said. "I was hoping if I told you my symptoms, you might diagnose something else—a disease you could cure. I take my medicine, but my case is difficult to control. I am not doing well. I am afraid."

I was embarrassed and disappointed, but most of all I felt sorry for him. I had been so euphoric about diagnosing my first case of myasthenia gravis that I had forgotten my concern for Mr. Thomas.

From that day to this, I guard against thinking of patients as interesting. Diseases are interesting. Patients are sick.

# 'I HAD A BABY SISTER BUT SHE ONLY LASTED ONE DAY'

## Susan C. M. Schrimshaw, Ph.D., and Daniel M. S. March, Ph.D.

"We love you, Elisabeth, we'll never forget you." Five-year-old Corey spoke these words to her sister, who had been born the night before and now lay dying because of severe congenital defects. Twenty-four hours earlier, if you had asked us if we thought a child should see a deformed, dying sibling, we would have been surprised that the question was even asked. During the sad 24 hours of Elisabeth's life, Corey taught us a great deal about our own feelings and about a child's capacity to handle illness and death.

The first indications of problems with the pregnancy came after Susan had amniocentesis. I was present for the procedure, and we both were thrilled to see our baby waving her hand on the ultrasound screen. We confidently waited to hear that everything was all right.

Everything was not all right. The geneticist had found two odd bits of extra chromosomes, something neither she nor any other geneticist she consulted had ever seen before. There was nothing on this in the medical literature either. Since the extra chromosomes were in only 8% of the cells examined, it was impossible to determine whether they were fetal in origin. Even if they were fetal cells, there was no way of knowing what phenotypic effect (if any) they would have. The finding was unsettling, but there did not seem to be sufficient evidence to justify interrupting the pregnancy. We told ourselves that at least we knew all the things that the baby did not have and hoped that everything was fine. We asked to know the baby's sex, and in late July, we told our 5-year-old daughter, Corey, that she would get a baby sister. Corey was not pleased: "You guys got it all wrong; I wanted a *brother*."

Corey is a strong, independent child, and it took a while to convince her that you have to take what you get in the baby department. We spoke of the fun of having a sister, of teaching her to do things, of having party dresses that matched, of being girls together. We chose the name Elisabeth Herriott, a composite of family names. We did all the things parents do to prepare a child for a sibling, and by fall Corey was eagerly awaiting "our baby."

In September, Corey started kindergarten and Susan went to bed. Frequent mild-to-moderate contractions had developed, cervical effacement had begun, and she had polyhydramnios, all conditions that make premature labor more likely. Sonography showed that Elisabeth appeared to be developing normally, but since Susan was at only 30 weeks' gestation, the obstetrician thought it best for her to spend most of her time at bed rest. Susan is a university professor who had always worked and traveled (sometimes with Corey). Suddenly she was unable to get up to make Corey dinner or watch her climb a tree. She and Corey could read and talk and draw together, but Corey would speak longingly of the time when Mother would "be normal again." At the same time, Elisabeth grew more active, and Corey delighted in feeling her sister's vigorous kicking and in singing lullabies to Susan's pregnant abdomen.

One Friday in November, Susan went to the hospital to have some of the excess amniotic fluid drawn off. It showed traces of meconium, evidence that the baby was not doing well. Since it was now only three weeks before Elisabeth was due and sonography showed that she was a big baby, the decision was made to induce birth. We had chosen an obstetrical group and a community hospital that encourage family-oriented birth and allow siblings at deliveries. Corey had asked if she could be present when Elisabeth "came out.'' We read and talked about birth with her and arranged for her to be present near the end of labor and for the delivery if everything seemed to be going well.

The amniotic sac was ruptured in the late afternoon, and by 7 PM, labor had progressed so far that we called our friend who was looking after Corey and suggested they leave for the hospital soon. It was a fast but uneventful labor until the baby's heart began to show bradycardia, a sign of fetal distress. The heart tones deteriorated rapidly, and Susan was told to push hard, fast, and continuously. I saw everything immediately—the color was wrong, she wasn't breathing, her lip and palate were cleft, her thumbs were elongated, and her ears were low-set. I felt like I had suddenly hit a brick wall. Our obstetrician gently told us that the baby had a cleft lip and palate and that it was possible that there were other problems as well. Elisabeth was whisked to the neonatal intensive care unit (ICU), and we sat quietly for a few moments, trying to absorb what had happened. Elisabeth was alive, but it was uncertain how long she would survive, or in what condition.

''Mommy?'' Corey's voice could be heard clearly from the hall. ''Mommy?'' I was still pale and shaky as I went out into the hall to intercept Corey. She was obviously afraid that something might happen to her mother. Moments later, she sat on Susan's bed as it was wheeled to another area of the room.

After a little while, she asked about her sister, and we told her that Elisabeth was very sick. ''I want to see her.'' Corey clearly expected to be dealt with in a straightforward way. Kate, our labor and delivery nurse, made a quick assessment of Corey's needs and abilities. She suggested that we let Corey see Elisabeth through the window in the hall some 15 feet from her bassinet so that the most obvious defects would not be too apparent. Corey looked for a moment, then said: ''Those wires on her look just like E.T.'s before he died. Is Elisabeth going to die?'' I told her all we knew at the time: ''Elisabeth is very sick and it is possible that she will die. We don't know yet how bad it is.''

Before I left, Susan and I went into the neonatal ICU with Jeff, our pediatrician, and saw Elisabeth. Since my research is on seizure disorders and Susan's is on childbirth, we both knew right away how much was wrong. Jeff told us he doubted Elisabeth would survive the night. Together, we took inventory of her problems, which included an enlarged fontanelle, congenital cataracts, and cardiac and respiratory irregularities in addition to the features I had observed at delivery. Later that night, Susan had her bed wheeled into the ICU next to Elisabeth's bassinet, and the two of them shared some quiet hours.

On Saturday morning, Elisabeth was still alive and Corey insisted on seeing her. "She wasn't made right, Corey. She's going to die." "I want to see Elisabeth." "We'll see what we can arrange, Corey, but her face will look strange; it didn't come together right." Quietly, sadly, we talked about what Elisabeth looked like, why she would die, and how we felt.

That afternoon, Corey and I met Susan in the neonatal ICU. Corey was given a child-sized cover gown, and we entered the small room where Elisabeth now was the sole occupant. The nurses stayed discreetly back, just outside the door, as we approached Elisabeth. Corey stood on Susan's wheelchair and looked at Elisabeth, now free of wires and tubes. "Ooo, gross!" she said as she saw her sister's face. She turned to Susan. "Can I touch her?" Susan nodded. Corey reached inside the bassinet and began to stroke Elisabeth's bare arm. "Her skin is so soft! Look, she has curly red hair! It's soft, too!" Corey turned again to Susan and said tearfully, "She's going to die." Turning back to Elisabeth, Corey began to talk to her. "Your skin is so soft, Elisabeth. I wish you didn't have to die. We love you." Elisabeth began to move her arms and legs in response to Corey's voice and touch. Corey turned around with an expression of delight on her face. "She loves me! She knows I'm here!" For a long time, Corey stroked and talked with Elisabeth, holding her hand, caressing her hair. Finally, it was time to go. Corey repeated: "We love you, Elisabeth.

We'll never forget you. We'll never forget you." Behind Corey, we sat in stunned silence. Behind us, some of the nurses wiped tears from their eyes. How did Corey know to say hello, I love you, and good-bye to her dying sister?

Corey didn't want to leave. "I want to stay with Elisabeth. I want to see Elisabeth die." We were shocked. See Elisabeth die? How morbid! "No, Corey, we can't do that. For one thing, we don't know when she will die, how long it will take."

At home that night, as Susan was reading Corey a bedtime story, the telephone rang. It was Jeff. "Elisabeth died a few minutes ago, at 8:30. I'm sorry." We all cried together, numb, sad, but also relieved that Elisabeth's discomfort had ended. A few minutes later the telephone rang again. Elisabeth's pediatric nurse called to say that she had been with Elisabeth as she died, had stroked her and talked to her, and that she had let go peacefully. Suddenly, we regretted that we hadn't been there with her and said to ourselves, "Corey was right; we should have been there when she died."

On Sunday morning, the hospital asked me to come in to sign the death certificate and make arrangements for an autopsy. Corey insisted on going. "I want to see Elisabeth dead." We didn't know how to react to this but decided she could at least go with me to sign the papers. At the hospital, Corey bided her time. She waited until we were in the head nurse's office. "I want to see my sister dead."

The head nurse asked Corey a few questions, then spoke to me. "I just took a course on children and death. I think she should see Elisabeth. I'm more concerned about how you will hold up than I am with her."

The nurse made arrangements to see Elisabeth in a small room adjacent to the hospital morgue. She told us that Elisabeth was somewhat blotchy and purple. Corey didn't seem to be affected by the description. She simply wanted to see for herself.

Elisabeth was wrapped in a blanket and set on a shelf in the small room. Corey was sad and fascinated at once. She

reviewed the physical deformities apparent to her and reminded herself that Elisabeth had other problems she
couldn't see that couldn't be fixed. She touched Elisabeth
several times, repeating that she would never be forgotten,
that it was very sad that she had died, and how much she
loved her. After several minutes we left the room, thanked
the nurse, and went home.

In the weeks that followed, we found that allowing Corey
to take the lead in what she needed to do with Elisabeth
was more valuable than we ever could have predicted. There
were no nightmares about a deformed baby; the reality had
been seen and acknowledged. The misshapen face was only
one feature. Elisabeth also had features to love like her soft
skin and hair and responsiveness to Corey. We did not have
to conceal our grief from Corey but could share it. Each of
us spoke up when we were sad, to be comforted by one of
the others. At grace one day, Corey said, "God, we are
grateful for Elisabeth, but we are not grateful for what happened to her."

Corey also expressed anger, a normal reaction, but sometimes distressingly sudden. We were very upset when a
pregnant friend paid a condolence call, only to be greeted
at the front door by a wordless Corey, who took one look
at her abdomen and punched it. We talked to Corey about
hurt and angry feelings that were real and important but
could not be expressed through violence. It got better. A
few weeks later, Corey and Susan saw a friend with a baby
who had soft, curly red hair. Corey turned away quickly,
and Susan asked how she felt. "I feel jealous" was the
reply. Words had replaced blows. Corey also voiced feelings
of guilt that perhaps a cold Susan caught from her in October had hurt Elisabeth. We tried to convey to Corey that
Elisabeth's problems had developed very early and that a
cold in October could not have caused them.

We will probably never know what caused the genetic
anomalies. Our own tissue culture results were normal.
Since Elisabeth was the first baby identified with that particular chromosome pattern, if it is seen again after amni-

ocentesis a couple can be told what the consequences are likely to be. With enthusiastic support from Corey and excellent odds for a normal baby, we will try again. Corey has plenty of suggestions for the next baby: "How about twins? Then if something happens, we'll still have one."

A question might be raised about how much Corey really understood about the permanence of death. We have always been very straightforward with Corey. She was 2 years old when our pet cat died. She watched us bury the cat, then asked when she would come out again. When we said she wouldn't, Corey wanted to know why we couldn't take her to the doctor and get her fixed. By the time her great-grandmother died, Corey was almost 4 years old and understood that death was irrevocable.

Despite experience with more "normal" deaths, when faced with the hypothetical question of how to handle a child's involvement in the birth and death of a sibling, we probably would have given the conventional answers: a child should be told the truth gently but protected from "traumatic" sights and experiences. Corey taught us a lot about her abilities to handle death, about children's perception of life and death, about their needs, and about ourselves and our feelings. She taught us to listen to children more carefully. As she put it later: "When my baby sister was born my daddy didn't know how to love her, but I showed him."

# 'DADDY'

## William H. Hunter, M.D.

Back in 1953 I had just begun my practice in the small town of Clemson at the foot of the Blue Ridge Mountains in South Carolina. In the beginning I spent a lot of time reading medical journals and waiting for the local people to find out was in town.

One August evening near dusk, my wife, Jane, and I were sitting in the swing when two farmers approached the porch and asked: "You the new doctor?" I nodded.

"Well, Doc, Daddy's down and sick and the doctor we called isn't treating him right."

"What's the matter?"

"This here doctor wants to put Daddy in the hospital."

I asked what he'd been treating him for.

"He hadn't been treating him for nothin'. Last time Daddy had a doctor was in '33, when he fell out of the loft and broke his leg."

"Well, what did the doctor say was the matter?" I asked.

"He said Daddy was havin' a heart attack, and damned if he was gonna treat him at home. He wanted to take him down to the hospital in Anderson, Doc. That's 20 miles away. Are you comin' to see him or we just gonna stand here and talk?"

So, after going by my office and getting my new ECG machine that had never been used on a sick patient, I fol-

lowed their truck up through the rolling hills toward the foo
of the mountains.

This was the most beautiful country in the world, covered
with small and middle-sized farms inhabited by very independent people. They'd come from Celtic stock and had
been there since they drove out the Cherokee in 1781 (after
the Indians came out for King George). They were fiercely
loyal to each other, shared a common dislike for revenuers,
voted Republican in a Democratic state, and yet were the
most hospitable people I'd ever met. Pickens County, South
Carolina, had produced more congressional Medal of Honor
recipients than any other in the United States, and while
there's no record, they probably had more court-martialings
as well.

"Daddy," whom I was going to see, turned out to be the
patriarch of this part of the country. When we arrived, there
were about 50 people standing around under the white oaks.
Daddy raised himself from his bed, gasping a bit. He gave
me a look that said: "Is this the best those boys could do?
Guess I'll just have to put up with him."

He was 76 years old. The ECG confirmed a myocardial
infarction with numerous PVCs, and there were wet rales
in both lung bases. I was six weeks out of what I thought
was a good internship in one of the best teaching hospitals
in the Carolinas, but I wasn't prepared for this. My looks
must have betrayed me (Celtic types read a lot into looks),
because Daddy gasped: "Doc, I was born in this house,
lived here all my life, and I'm gonna die in this house. You
just do the best you can."

I sent for an oxygen tank and sent Jane to the hospital for
heparin. I used mercuhydrin intravenously and sat by his
bed poking nitroglycerin into him and injecting Demerol
until about 1 AM, when he was finally free of pain and his
lungs began to clear. I went back out on the porch for some
fresh air and saw that more than 100 people had gathered
under the trees. When I left at sunrise, many of them were
still there.

I'm sure, deep down, that Daddy's recovery had more to

do with his tough constitution, but I got the credit. There's never been a want of patients in my practice since then. And from that time, I was always invited to their family reunions, where the preacher would sit on one side of Daddy and I sat on the other.

Triage *is a word you won't find in many dictionaries, but doctors use it all the time, even though most of them don't know where it comes from.* Tree-ahj, *with the accent on the first syllable, means to direct patients to an appropriate area for medical care. The word is used both as a verb and as a noun, an actual place where such decisions are made.*

*In large metropolitan emergency rooms, disaster areas, and other emergency situations, doctors will set up an area to examine patients quickly and then will make rapid decisions where the patients should be taken for further, more comprehensive treatment.*

*Few know that the term was first used by Napoleon's Surgeon General in an attempt to deal with the massive number of casualties suffered by the French troops during the Napoleonic Wars. He decided to divide the wounded into three groups (hence the term* triage*): those whose wounds were so slight that they were not in need of immediate medical attention, those whose injuries were so severe that medical care would be of no use, and last, those who would benefit from what little medicine had to offer at the turn of the 19th century.*

*Physicians have always been involved when man waged war with his fellow man. In fact, the Surgeon General of the United States retains that title from the early days of military medicine. The Surgeon General is not only head of the US Public Health Service but Commander-in-Chief of the Commissioned Corps, part of the Uniformed Services. That is why you will see him decked out in his uniform—a naval uniform, because the Public Health Service started out as part of the US Navy in 1798. All Commissioned Corps officers carry a military rank, and many of the doctors and nurses who work at the Centers for Disease Control (CDC)*

*in Atlanta, Georgia, the National Institutes of Health in Be-
thesda, Maryland, the Food and Drug Administration in
Washington, DC, and the other venues of the Public Health
Service carry a military commission—and can be called up
without notice to serve in times of national crisis.*

*Although I was an infectious disease specialist in the Ep-
idemic Intelligence Service at the CDC in 1980, I carried
the designated title of senior assistant surgeon in the Public
Health Service, and the rank of lieutenant commander,
equivalent to a major in the Army.*

*In May 1980, during the exodus from Cuba's Mariel Har-
bor, I was confronted with that rank for the first time. I was
asked to be medical director of screening for the 20,000
Cuban refugees who had been abruptly airlifted into Fort
Chaffee, Arkansas. We had in short order to examine the
men, women, and children for any contagious diseases as
well as to contend with any medical problems that were
bound to develop when that many people were suddenly
thrown together.*

*I and my staff had to battle the blistering heat of an over-
crowded camp, a massive outbreak of food poisoning, and
an epidemic of spinal meningitis, all of us wearing olive
drab Army fatigues and I with gold oak-leaf clusters on my
shoulders and a caduceus (the snake-entwined staff of medicine) on my collar. While US Army Green Berets in their
camouflage uniforms paraded around the barbed wire with
bayoneted M-16s, I tried with my rudimentary Spanish to
establish some kind of rapport with a campful of tired and
frightened strangers.*

*Although I've never had to serve in actual wartime, those
of my colleagues who have will attest to the intensity of the
exposure and the changes they have undergone because of
the experience. There are hazards to being a noncombatant
in areas of conflict—there are also rewards.*

B.B.D.

# A Wet Mouse

## Jack C. Redman, M.D.

It was summer in the Mekong Delta. Miles of rice paddies, crisscrossed by canals, lay under humid, motionless air. Midday temperatures were 110 degrees. I was in the provincial hospital in Bac Lieu, South Vietnam, located 120 miles southwest of Saigon, on the southeastern coast of the war-torn country. Not far to the west lay the U Minh forest, sanctuary of the Viet Cong.

I had flown to Vietnam the month before. I was one of a group of the American Medical Association's Volunteer Physicians for Vietnam. Dr. Meritt Stark, a Denver pediatrician, and I had been assigned to go to Bac Lieu, a city of 60,000 people. He was a pediatrician and I was a surgeon. We were to work with the Vietnamese *chef du medicin* Dr. Nguyen Thu Vinh and the US Army doctors of the 51st Advisory Team. The only American troops in Bac Lieu, the officers and men of the 51st were advisors to the 21st Division of the Army of the Republic of Vietnam.

The hospital consisted mostly of a cluster of early-1900s French-built, tile-roofed structures. Facilities were primitive, but the excellent staff of American Army physicians, nurses, and medical technicians showed us how to make the most out of what we had. Only the most basic laboratory tests were possible. Physicians had to rely mostly on their own best judgment in making diagnoses and carrying out treatment.

In surgery we had fine instruments and materials, provided by the United States. The Army doctors and Dr. Vinh were fine physicians and surgeons whose individual skills far outweighed the adversities of their type of practice.

Women and children relatives of patients moved in with the patients many times, sleeping under the beds or in them with the patients. The women cooked food on little charcoal stoves outside the buildings. Goats, pigs, and oxen roamed the grounds. There was one goat that liked to stand in the window of the administration building and a pig with a penchant for wandering into the postoperative surgical building. A few buildings had no electricity, making nighttime candlelight visits there a necessity.

I was eating in the Army mess hall one noon when a young Vietnamese woman ran in from the emergency building and told me to come quickly to see a baby who was dying. Despite all the anguish the Vietnamese people had seen during the war, a sick baby still evoked feelings of desperation. We ran to the emergency ward and found a young mother holding her baby. The little boy couldn't have been 10 months old. He was so sick he couldn't cry. He was burning up with fever and dry as a bone, his lips cracked and bleeding. His breathing was erratic.

As I bent over to examine his ears, nose, and throat, I smelled something strange, like nothing I had ever smelled before. No, I *had* smelled it before, but where? It smelled like a wet mouse. A wet mouse? I *had* smelled it, in Denver, 17 years ago. . . .

I was a senior at the University of Colorado School of Medicine. One afternoon Dr. Leo Flax took our pediatrics clerkship group to the contagion unit of Denver General Hospital and showed us two young brothers who had diphtheria. He told us that we would probably never again see a case of diphtheria, so he wanted us to see these two cases and to smell the "wet mouse" odor of a diphtheritic membrane. "Once you've smelled it," he said, "you'll never forget it. . . ."

Meritt arrived back from the orphanage across the canal, where he had been making his weekly rounds. He agreed with my diagnosis. Before an IV could be started, the baby died. Meritt made a call to USAID (US Agency for International Development) headquarters in Saigon, and they had diphtheria antitoxin to us within three hours. Meritt inoculated all of the baby's contacts. Two days later, throat cultures confirmed what Dr. Flax had taught me to recognize 17 years before, half a world away. A raging epidemic was stopped in 1967, in the Mekong Delta, by a wet mouse.


# CLAYMORE CLARA

## Kirk V. Cammack, M.D.

Although it is over 15 years since I left Vietnam, the memory of one of my Vietnamese patients continues to haunt me. I was one of the physicians who, under the auspices of the American Medical Association, volunteered for two months' medical service to Vietnamese civilians.

Claymore Clara was a Viet Cong patient I treated at the Provincial Hospital in Nha Trang, South Vietnam. She had been nicknamed Claymore Clara by one of the nurses. Once most of the Viet Cong realized that we were not going to eat their liver, drink their blood, or steal their children (as they had been propagandized to believe), they became quite appreciative of our care. But not Claymore Clara.

Her Viet Cong group had been caught by the Green Berets laying Claymore mines around the Cam Rhan Bay area, and by the time the action was over, Clara was the only survivor. She had been crippled by an M-16 high-velocity missile that had pulverized her right femur. Claymore Clara's face was darkly beautiful, yet she was a surly, snarling 17-year-old who reminded me of the juvenile delinquents I had treated in inner-city hospitals in the United States. No matter what the staff did to try to win her over she remained indifferent to our overtures and at times was downright hostile.

One day, I came to her cot to check her infected wound through the cast on her leg (all the wounds in Vietnam seemed to be infected). She was lying on her side with one hand under her head; the other hand clutched her elbow. She was underweight and her dainty hands seemed large, like the hands of slum children I had treated. Her skeleton was outlined sharply under starvation flesh. No one had ever come to visit her and no relative had followed Claymore Clara to the hospital to care for her or feed her. Even though we had no central kitchen at the hospital she must have been getting some food, because she was alive, although thin. I had been bringing her candy and potato chips almost every day and, although she never acknowledged the gifts, they were never at her bedside the next time I came. This did not mean necessarily that she was eating them; they might be going to a Viet Cong soldier or perhaps were stolen by the other people in the ward.

"How are you, Clara?" I asked. She stared back at me.

I picked up a pair of sharp surgical scissors and worked her dressings. I could feel the tenseness of her body and I wondered if she could ever forgive or forget. "You really hate me, don't you, honey?" I asked softly.

I didn't expect a return smile or comment, nor did I get one. I kept up the chatter in English with a few clumsy Vietnamese words thrown in. "Don't worry, we will have you out of here before too long and then you can go back to laying more Claymore mines. That's what you plan to do, isn't it?''

No response.

By this time I had the dressing off the wound and noted with satisfaction that the infection was clearing. I was absorbed in checking the wound and did not notice her raise her head and look at the instrument tray, nor was I aware of any stealthy movement. The first indication that something was happening was when, with a sudden piercing scream, she made her play. Out of the corner of my eye I saw her stick-like arm rapidly descending, the thin hand gripping sharp scissors. I yelled in surprise, shoved away the bed, and fell to the floor, the scissors barely missing my neck. From the floor, I looked up at her. Her face was impassive, her eyes remained as they had been, unchanged, expressing consummate hatred. She slowly relaxed the grip on the scissors and they dropped to the floor. She placed her right hand under her head again, gripping the elbow with the other hand as before, and looked at me as if nothing had happened. The other patients in the ward watched impassively. Had they noticed what she was doing? Why didn't they warn me? There was complete silence. I picked myself up just as two nurses came rushing into the ward.

''What's going on here?'' one demanded.

''Oh,'' I said, ''Clara was just showing me how to use these scissors and was expressing her gratitude for my care.''

Until the last week of my time in Vietnam, Clara remained hostile. Then something happened that illustrated the complete unreality of that war. The Green Beret who had wounded Claymore Clara and killed her companions came to visit her. His accent reflected that he was probably from a large Eastern city. He was a wiry, tough, cocky Italian with a heavily lined face. His nose had been broken several times and his two front teeth were jagged. About the only sign of softness and tenderness was in his eyes, warm large eyes outlined by long dark lashes. He was accompanied by an interpreter and another Green Beret, a tall black man with huge shoulders, who looked like he could handle himself in any physical situation. Both men had a deep, solid friendship that came from sharing many close calls with death. Both wore the Montagnard Honorary gold bracelets on their wrists, a symbol that they had been made blood brothers with the mountain tribes of Vietnam.

When she saw them approaching, Clara shrank back as far as the confines of her cot would permit. When she could retreat no farther she tensed her body in an attack crouch and waited for a possible coup de grace. You could tell that she believed these American devils were capable of any atrocity. The hate in her eyes was her only weapon.

The soldier looked down at his victim, his eyes full of tears. He squatted beside her bed, not ignoring her attempts to murder him with her eyes. He began to talk softly to her. No one, except the interpreter who squatted beside the soldier and also spoke in soft tones, would ever know what the American sergeant said that day. But whatever was said had a definite effect. Claymore Clara relaxed, and suddenly, she started to cry and to speak so rapidly that the interpreter could not keep up. When she finished her story she was exhausted and too drained even for tears. The American soldier took 300 piastres from his pocket and gave them to her, and with trembling voice said, "I will see what I can do to get your watch and ring back, Clara." He touched her on the shoulder, and smiling, turned and marched from the ward followed by his buddy and the interpreter.

Outside the ward the Green Beret repeated her story to me.

Clara's village was near a river and that river was spanned by a bridge that was essential for the farmers' transportation in the area. There had been frequent interruptions in Clara's family activities because of the bridge. When Clara was quite young, the Viet Minh would come to the village and draft her father and brothers to blow up the bridge. After they had gone, within a week or so, the French troops would show up and draft them to replace the bridge.

When she was 16 the Viet Cong recruiters came to the

village where Clara lived. Clara was excited by the promises of adventure, and she was particularly stirred by a chance to leave the village, but she was devoted to her family and refused to accept the call to go. But "Charlie" got rough and pointed his gun at her parents, threatening to kill them if she did not go with them. Claymore Clara became a Viet Cong that day.

During the early Viet Cong indoctrination, Clara was the captain's chattel, which to her was sometimes exciting and at least different. It was also away from the hated bridge. She was subjected to constant indoctrination about the Americans and the war. Even though she had been constantly violated by the Viet Cong, she focused her hatred on Americans. To Clara, any white man was an American, a foreign white devil.

Clara rose through the ranks until she became a fighter. She became an expert at laying Claymore mines, which she was doing when the Green Berets surprised her party at Cam Rhan Bay. After she was wounded by the Americans she was turned over to the South Vietnamese for transportation to a hospital. At this time her sole possessions were a ring, a $5 watch, and 300 piastres, which the South Vietnamese promptly took from her and delivered her to the Provincial Hospital at Nha Trang.

Within a few days of the incident in the ward I left Vietnam to return to the United States. Before I left, I went to the PX and bought Clara some Chanel No. 5. She managed a hint of a smile as I gave her the perfume but would not let me take her hand. Tears came to my eyes and I said, "I am sorry, Clara, I really am." I turned and left the hospital for the last time.

# DEAR JOHN

## David L. Anders, M.D.

Dear John,

Kenya and I had dinner with Lisa last night. She seems to be making the adjustment to being a single parent fairly well. Some people may think I'm crazy to be writing you this letter, but I have my reasons. You and I have always understood each other—more like brothers really—as we went through grade school and high school and being roommates at college and medical school. I never told you that one of the greatest honors in my life was being best man when you married Lisa. But things change.

I recently read that 1,187,000 couples were divorced in 1985. Why does divorce have to happen? I don't suppose those 1,187,000 couples understand why. I don't imagine you understand why. I don't understand why. I guess it's too late to do much for the "class of 1985," but if those currently considering divorce could talk with you or with Lisa I wonder if they wouldn't give it another chance.

As I said, Lisa is doing OK. She has become fiercely independent in some ways—learned how to paint the house, strip the oak floors, buy a car. Coping in other areas may take more time than the four years she has had to learn: PTA meetings alone, the dating scene. Will's birthdays.

It seems like just last week that I was on call as a house officer when you called so late at night to tell me about your brand-new baby. Like most 4-year-olds, Will now encounters new experiences with almost every step he takes. I took him to his first football game a few weeks ago. It was just your basic high school game to me, between two teams I knew very little about, but for Will it was a life event—his first exposure to the idea of Musketeers vs Wild Cats, marching bands, cheerleaders, banners, pom-poms, school colors, kickoffs, and field goals. And last night at dinner I kept him entertained while Kenya and Lisa talked. He asked me if I would be his daddy—but he deserves better than me. He deserves you.

But then there are a lot of kids who deserve better, more than just a father on the weekends. It's ironic that the hard work and long hours that so many fathers invest so their children will "have things better" actually wind up taking away from quality family time at best—or result in parents who no longer feel a reason or desire to be married to each other at worst. And the casualties of the parents' wars are the Innocents.

Seeing what you have lost made my marriage with Kenya seem all the more treasured. John, I wish there were some way, any way I could get you and Lisa and Will back together—you know I would. But I can't. What happened in Beirut can never be changed. Fortunately for those of us left here, some things can.

We all miss you,<br>
David

John Rice Hudson, M.D., was assigned to care for the US Marines stationed in Beirut, Lebanon, at the time of the bombing of the military barracks there in October 1983. He is survived by his widow, Lisa, and his son, Will.

# COMMAND PERFORMANCE

## Emanuel Rubin, M.D.

Before I began my training in pathology, I worked for a short time as a general practitioner in the Catskill Mountains of New York, near my home in the small village of Liberty. The area was the site of numerous resort hotels and summer camps, among which were a few that were owned by Chasidic Jews from Brooklyn. These are Jews who belong to deeply religious (indeed, ultraorthodox) sects, dress in distinctive and antique black garb, and blend traditional piety with fervent mysticism. Being a moderately traditional if not overly pious Jew, I related well to the occasional Chasidic patient.

Close to midnight on a Friday evening I received an urgent call from a Chasidic hotel that some catastrophe had overtaken the Rabbi (their spiritual and secular leader) and that I must immediately be on my way to save him. I negotiated ten miles of dark, twisting mountain roads in less than 15 minutes, only to be greeted by a shower of stones from a group of children (up past their bedtime) who were expressing their disapproval of driving on the Sabbath. I disregarded the children, the stones, and the cracked window and skidded up to the main entrance.

As I rushed into the lobby, I saw at the far end of the room, through the crowd of black hats, beards, and agitated women, a sofa on which reclined a figure. Even without approaching further, it was clear to me from a distance that

103

the Rabbi was dead. Later I learned that he had had a history of heart disease, and I surmise that he suffered an acute myocardial infarction. I made my way through the wailing women and anxious men, took out my stethoscope, and placed it over the heart. The silence in the earpieces was matched by a similar quiet that had befallen my audience of perhaps 100. I realized that, considering the news I was about to impart, I should make some gestures; I took the pulse, listened again to various parts of the chest, and examined the eyes. The body was already cooling when I turned to the Chasidim and said, "I am sorry to tell you that the Rabbi has passed on." As I turned to close my bag and put on my jacket, a crescendo of hysterical weeping filled the room, and several women fainted. I began to make my way to the door, when a group of elders—a committee, if you will—asked me to stay for a moment. Their spokesman, a patriarch with a magnificent white beard and piercing dark eyes, explained to me that the Rabbi was a very holy man, that he embodied all their hopes and ideals, and that both they and the Almighty would be eternally grateful if I would try to "do something" to revive the Rabbi. Who knows what wonders might be achieved today by an aggressive resuscitation team, but on that evening in 1958 I was sure that the Rabbi had already passed through the portals of heaven. Yet with 200 Old Testament eyes fixed on me, I had to, at the very least, provide an opportunity for God to work a miracle.

With deliberate flourish, I withdrew a large syringe from my bag, attached it to a long spinal needle (why on earth did I carry it around?), and filled it with the first fluid that came into my hand. My audience gasped as I plunged the needle into the precordial area and injected the fluid. After waiting a minute I withdrew the syringe and listened with my stethoscope for an interminable moment. I finally turned to the elders and told them that the most drastic treatment known to medicine had been ineffective and that I had done my best, but the Lord had simply not restored the Rabbi. No physician has ever been thanked more sincerely, and as

I left, only a soft, plaintive murmur accompanied me to my car.

Did I lie? Was I dishonest? Did I act out a charade? Would Sisela Bok approve? Would Ralph Nader chastise me? I can only say that although I did nothing for the Rabbi, his followers *felt* better because they believed that I had made extraordinary efforts and that, for his own good reasons, God had merely seen fit not to intervene. I felt better too.

# PREPARATION

## Hugh F. Johnston, M.D.

My teachers in medical school were responsible people who realized that students often have difficulty dealing with the issues of death and dying. Thus, we had to read several papers and books on the subject and we all attended discussion groups. In these groups we talked a great deal about death. We discussed terminal illness, euthanasia, how we experienced death in our families, and even how we felt about our own eventual death. These groups met weekly for a whole semester, and when all of this scholarly work was done, we had a simple pass-fail essay examination. At the time it all seemed quite sensible and the course left us with that satisfying feeling of having reasonably mastered another subject. A year later, on the wards, I met Mr. P.

He was a typical veteran, a middle-aged bachelor with no known family. He had come in very short of breath with almost constant hemoptysis—a legacy of 30 years of smoking. There was little we could do for him, since he had been through the whole gamut of surgery, chemotherapy, and radiation. Yet, as usual, the tumor in his lung continued to grow. He spent the first two days in the hospital sitting up in bed gasping for air, coughing up bits of blood-tinged sputum. We all tried to comfort him as much as possible and he was always very appreciative. But he knew the end was coming soon and sometimes during a coughing fit, he would choke badly and I could see terror in his eyes. I stopped by his room as often as I could to check on him and ask how he was doing. He would breathlessly reply "Not good" and shake his head.

On the third day of hospitalization a nurse burst into the chart-room yelling for us to come quickly because Mr. P. was in trouble. We ran to his bed and found him sitting up with a washbasin in his lap already half full of dark, slithery clots. He was struggling terribly—drowning in his own blood. His face was deep purple and his eyes bulged out in stark terror. As the bleeding became worse, so did the struggle. There was less and less real breathing but more awful choking. Violently he would attempt to take a breath only to have it cut short by choking and coughing. Great quantities of blood bubbled out through his mouth and nose, ran down his chin, and dribbled into his lap. He would then cough explosively, splattering us with blood. The sound was horrifying, like someone screaming under water. Meanwhile, the nurse and I were trying to help as best we could. I tried to keep the oxygen mask close yet emptied of blood; she tried to help him clear the bigger pieces from his mouth and throat. The intern was frantically working the phone trying to get some help. But it was hopeless; the blood just kept coming and the scene became more macabre. A beard of stringy blood clots swung heavily from the man's chin and nose. Between coughing spells he rocked back and forth, gasping, "Oh please, oh please."

Suddenly it was quiet; it must have been a big clot. His mouth was open and his chest was heaving but no air was moving. He looked at each of us in turn, pleading with his eyes. We pounded him on the back but nothing helped. Still, he kept straining desperately to breathe, opening and closing his mouth like some strange, soundless imitation of a fish. During what seemed like an eternity he silently struggled. Finally his eyelids began to sag and we gently eased him back in the bed. He continued to make feeble respiratory attempts as he turned bluish gray. Then he had a seizure and lay there, twitching and quivering with the bed making little squeaks as if to keep time. It was a long time before that too finally stopped.

No one moved. The nurse looked stupidly blank, covered with blood. The intern was still holding the phone, weeping. I thought about my class on death and dying. They hadn't considered a terrified, helpless old man dying a horrible, gory, painful death. The books, the papers, the discussion groups—all seemed irrelevant and far away. But close at hand was fear, sadness, and futility.

# THE 'TERRIBLE' QUESTION

## Stanley M. Bierman, M.D.

The wide-eyed and fearful expression on the face of the 68-year-old, heavy-set Russian immigrant did not betray any hidden secret as she sat across from my office desk while I read the hand-scribed physician's prescription, on which was written: ''Please examine Mrs. G. for a 1:16 serologic test for syphilis. It is probably a biologic false-positive test.''

Mrs. G. appeared worn and tired, although her graying hair was covered with a brightly colored babushka. Her stout physical habitus and plain, though not unattractive, appearance were strikingly similar to those of my own grand-mother, who had died during my childhood. Both were poor, unschooled Russian peasants who, despite their humble origins, maintained a special dignity in their bearing and demeanor.

Given the fact that my grandmother had fled Russian pogroms and my grandfather came to America to avoid conscription into the Czar's army, there was an instinctive identification with, and special consideration extended toward, the Russian-Jewish families and foreign émigrés who frequented my dermatology practice. Mrs. G. had come to this country in 1979 as part of a government policy to permit Russian Jews to immigrate to the United States. In halting English, punctuated by both Russian and Yiddish, Mrs. G. told me that she could not understand how she could have acquired this "gishlect" (terrible) disease. In a gentle manner I explained that sometimes the test result was positive for reasons other than syphilis, such as recent viral infections, immunizations, autoimmune disease, or merely as a natural finding in aging populations. My slow and careful scientific explanations were not apparently fully understood, or lost on the patient, for her bewilderment and confusion seemed unchanged.

I next explained to Mrs. G. that as part of a careful history I was required to ask certain questions of a personal nature that had bearing on the blood tests. I apologized in advance for any embarrassment she might experience.

"How long have you been married?" I inquired. "Fofzig [50] years," she responded. My reply, "Mazeltov," was quietly acknowledged by a single nod of her head. "Have you always been . . . ?" I hesitated, searching for an appropriate word. The pause was not lost on the patient. "Have you always been faithful to your husband?"

The patient's right hand was flung to her chest to cover her heart. Tears welled in her eyes as she haltingly answered in a quivering voice filled with both emotion and sincerity: "I have always been faithful to my husband." I felt no further need to question her virtue, but did carefully continue.

I next gently inquired as to when she had last had sexual intercourse with her husband. I learned that her husband had suffered a stroke four years previously, which along with his diabetes had rendered him impotent. Despite my instincts to drop the sensitive issue of her fidelity lest I be perceived as being too harsh in my interrogation, I once again inquired, "Are you *absolutely* certain that you have been faithful to your husband?" With the same gesture of her hand over her heart, she replied that in God's name she had been faithful.

I was about to embark on other questions relating to a biologic false-positive test result for syphilis but chose to pause for a moment's reflection. I was struck both by my discomfort in the interview and by the seeming incongruity of confronting an elderly, Jewish, foreign-born patient with social and moral questions better suited for a parish priest at a Catholic confessional. It was at that moment that I was struck with a revelation that had not heretofore been addressed. An important, if not terrible, question came to mind to ask of my patient. "Have you ever . . ." I quietly began. "Have you ever been sexually assaulted?" Mrs. G. looked at me with a frozen expression, much like the still frame at the end of a sad motion picture. A very long moment passed, after which she threw her hands over her eyes and began to sob uncontrollably.

The poignant story then unfolded as the patient painfully revealed her terrible secret. At no time following the brutal rape some four years previously had she ever confided this experience to a soul. Her embarrassment and humiliation were such that she never shared the fact of her rape with her husband, children, friends, or even her personal physician. How could she? How could an immigrant new to this country expl. n in her halting English the fact of her sexual assault to the police? In her mind, the police (Soviet, that is) were to be feared and not trusted. She kept her silence, and in her mind and heart she maintained the belief that she *was* faithful to her husband of 50 years. Yet she could not lie to me when confronted with my "terrible" question.

A definitive treatment program for latent syphilis was in-
stituted, and during the several follow-up visits in the office
she explained to me that the past four years had been a
nightmare for her. She was sick most of the time with head-
aches, stomachaches, high blood pressure, and endless so-
matic complaints emanating from the psychological trauma
of that tragic night. The dark secret of her rape that led to
these psychosomatic complaints was never revealed to her
physician.

When Mrs. G.'s treatment was completed I explained that
it would be necessary to see her in follow-up in three months
to repeat the blood tests. She observed that she already could
not pay my medical bills, but I explained that I was pleased
to extend professional services without charge.

The following day when I arrived at work I found a gift
at my office front door wrapped in a simple brown grocery
bag. Inside was an inexpensive silver-plated serving tray
that Mrs. G. must surely have brought from Russia. Carefully arranged in a geometric pattern on the tray were 20
crunchy pieces of home-baked apple strudel. Layers of wafer-
thin pie crusts enclosed delectable cinnamon-flavored
cooked apple slices that had been rolled in honey, raisins,
and walnuts.

Until that lovely moment, another great Russian lady—
my great-aunt Minnie—held title to the world's greatest apple strudel. It was the best dessert I ever had.

# MILES

## William M. Tierney, M.D.

I grin at the thought of how my habit of putting several miles of road beneath my feet every couple of days must appear to others, especially now as I pull on a pair of running shorts and a light jersey to face the first freezing weather of the winter season. Under a gray sky promising snow, I face into the wind as it whispers and growls across the Indiana farmland and turn on to a deserted country road.

In reality, I run in a cloud of memories of failures, of lost lives and abandoned hopes. As I run, I remember too well . . .

I remember Bradley, a young leukemic patient who had failed all standard and experimental chemotherapy, whose parents had lost their only other child to another malignancy, hating having her die in the confines of a sterile hospital, now only wanting their hopelessly ill son to die at home. I remember him in the hospital admitting room, the small purple lesions with black, necrotic centers on his extremities, his impossible fever, the obvious pseudomonal sepsis, his skin wet, pale, his eyes open too wide, the pupils too large, begging for release. His parents only wanted some relief, not a cure—we decided to give him a quick liter of saline, some narcotics, and whisked him home to die. Suddenly my heart feels heavy as I run, remembering the "stat" page to the admitting room, arriving there breathless, as I am now, seeing in the eyes of his parents that that death, too, had been stolen from them. Their kindness and thankfulness gall at me still. And I run.

I remember Judy, the second-grade schoolteacher in her 20s, pretty and ill, cyanotic in the ravages of postinfluenzal staphylococcal pneumonia. Day after day, disaster after disaster, I fought for each organ as it failed: the septic shock, the renal failure, the gastrointestinal bleeding, the gradual decline into delirium, the cardiac arrest, the resuscitation, the return of vital signs. Then came the months, the cachexia, the contractures. I remember the accusations of her parents with less pain and bitterness than Bradley's parents' understanding and forgiveness.

Then Bob, a kindly 55-year-old man whom I met in the coronary care unit of the Veterans Administration hospital, his third visit there for angina in two weeks. He had suffered three myocardial infarctions in two years. He showed me his work: he would hollow out blocks of Lucite with a motorized tool, delicate and patient work, and then paint the inside of the block with a minute brush to make roses so real as to astonish, frozen forever in plastic.

As I run, now sweating despite the biting of the wind as it swirls over the fence rows, I remember his acceptance of his death, foreseeing it unafraid, as I admonished him not to give up, that there was always hope; and his indulgent smile, without words. I was speaking to him of inconsequentials when he died, falling suddenly back against the pillows, surprising me by the speed with which he turned that sickly blue-gray. I remember the resuscitation as each piece of equipment failed, as I failed, and the long walk down the short corridor to tell his wife of his death. She knew, and she accepted. As I whipped myself before her, expounding my failures, her face mirrored those of Bradley's parents, showing kindness and forgiveness that hurt more than denigration.

I gather my dead about me as I run on this sunless November day across the Indiana farmland. I am running hard now, allowing the thoughts that all physicians cage deep within themselves to bubble to the surface and linger. I try to gain a hold on my place in all of this, and I find myself a part of the countryside, dead and barren, but within, beneath the frozen furrows, there lies a future, the next planting, the toil from which springs the next harvest. As from the windswept fields of November comes future plenty, so from the ashes of my memory, the losses and failures, come compassion for the suffering, passion for the living, and striving for what is right for my patient.

I head home now. The raw, wintry air roughens my throat as I run, but I run free. I have called up my shades once more and put them to rest. I am a man. I cannot place my talents above the lives of those whom I serve. I can only offer what I can, never enough, but all I have. I have neither beauty nor wisdom nor strength, only a heart that beats achingly against a frail chest, both on the road and in the passions of my art. Bradley, Judy, Bob, and all the others live on in me, making their way into my consciousness when they may, either on the backroads of Indiana or in the critical care waiting room. They are there, always there. Their lesson has been sobering, disquieting, and real. I listen when I can and run when I must.

# THE HARVARD WAY

## S. Walker, M.D.

There are times, every day, I need to swallow the urge to cry. And I need to keep telling myself that I'll be a good doctor. Maybe I'm just a product of the place where I was raised. People there were unassuming and usually kind at first meeting. Here there is no "Nice to meet you," there isn't even a chance to make a mistake. They assume you already have.

They have a way of making you feel worthless. Where they're coming from, or why they feel so superior, I don't know, but I think it's ironic. We work like slaves, get very little sleep, and have no formal didactic teaching on which to base our knowledge of the vast field of surgery. And if we don't perform well on standardized tests—there is no explaining—there is no help—there can be no suggestions. We just get degrading letters in our mailboxes about how poorly we have performed, encouraging us to get into a study program. Excuse me, but I thought that was supposed to be a part of residency!

This is supposed to be the mecca of medicine—in probably the country's most renowned medical city. You'd think they'd be proud to share their knowledge; after all, it's a "teaching institution." Well, they've "taught" me to feel afraid, worthless, ashamed, and often that I don't "deserve" to be a doctor. Physicians don't have the respect they once had. It's our own fault; we have dehumanized ourselves.

In two months I'll pack up and go home—by my own choice. I know that I am a good, caring doctor. But my self-worth and sense of competency have had to come from within. They've done everything they can to tear it down. This experience did *not* build character, strength, or "make a man" out of me. I am not and never will be one of the "good old boys." It has only given me many months of disappointment and sorrow. It is sad that people so bright and so famous have lost the ability to do a simple thing—to treat all people as equals. Someday we may *all* be in a situation where we can't handle the rejection anymore.

*"The Harvard Way" generated a good many letters to
JAMA. Among them were those who agreed with Dr. Walker's assessment of the often arduous and sometimes harsh
conditions that interns and residents speak about. Some
compared the treatment to that dished out by Marine drill
instructors. Others stated that the only way to "toughen
up" prospective physicians for the difficulties they will encounter in their careers and to screen out those who would
not make it was to put them through this type of training.*

*The Journal also received calls and letters from those as-
sociated with Harvard, protesting the singling out of that
institution. It should be clear that no single institution represents the best or the worst in medical training. The editor
of JAMA's "Letters to the Editor" section, Dr. Drummond
Rennie, stated that in publishing articles, The Journal allows its readers to reach their own conclusions concerning
the motives, balance, and accuracy of the pieces.*

*The following are excerpts from letters responding to
"The Harvard Way" as well as JAMA's editorial reply.*

B. B. D.

To the Editor:
I read with a great deal of sadness Dr. S. Walker's "The
Harvard Way." The feelings Dr. Walker expressed are a
stinging indictment of what I feel to be archaic attitudes in
graduate medical education. For some reason, physicians
who are supposed to epitomize compassion and sensitivity
tend to design training programs that are the antithesis of
such desirable attributes. Residents work long hours for little pay. They are expected to withstand severe psychological

and physical trials, and, instead of getting support and encouragement from their teachers, they receive stinging rebuke and are made to feel worthless and incompetent. I feel there is no reason for this. . . .

If residents are to be trained to meet the problems of the future, they must be exposed to role models who not only have superb medical skills, but also are physicians of exemplary strength of character, sensitivity, and compassion.

Bradford L. Walters, M.D.

To the Editor:
Dr. Walker described a phenomenon that is commonly known but seldom verbalized. There seems to be a strong relationship between academic achievement and insensitive behavior. Fortunately, there are many exceptions to this generalization. Those academicians who should be most concerned about this trend are often oblivious or indifferent. . . .

Perhaps Dr. Walker made a poor match. This can easily happen when applicants consider only the academic reputations of institutions. "The Harvard Way" is not unique to Harvard and certainly will continue. The most important lesson that can be learned from Dr. Walker's painful experience is that during the courtship between program and applicant, matching values and personal styles is as important as matching academic qualifications.

Jo Ellen Patterson, Ph.D.

To the Editor:
"The Harvard Way" is a telling description of how surgical residency programs are conducted at some "big-name" institutions. There are probably many other bright young men and women who bitterly drop out of surgical residencies because of the sort of inexcusable treatment Dr. Walker experienced.

One year ago, I was a medical student traveling around the country in search of a surgical residency. It appeared that the more prestigious the program, the more dissatisfied were the residents. . . .

After reading Dr. Walker's essay, I became even more confident that I had made the right choice in selecting my surgical residency program. . . . [It] is well respected; at the same time, it is strictly nonpyramidal, the on-call schedule is, at most, every third night, and the work is fairly distributed among all levels of residents. . . . What's more, the faculty is readily available for help and advice. As a result, there is a general sense of enthusiasm and camaraderie throughout the program.

Unlike Dr. Walker, I am experiencing the most exciting year of my life. Medical students who are selecting residency programs should learn to separate the name of the program from the quality of the program. Unfortunately, Dr. Walker had to learn the hard way.

Raymond L. Singer, M.D.

To the Editor:
I strenuously object to the unwarranted slur upon the Harvard Medical School and the many physicians associated with it in the essay entitled "The Harvard Way." . . . I have been a member of the faculty at the Harvard Medical School for ten years. The institution is full of dedicated physicians who are busy providing patient care, running teaching programs, and carrying out medical research—often "working like slaves and getting very little sleep," just like Dr. Walker. Hundreds of residents complete training at Harvard teaching hospitals each year and go on to pursue their medical careers, having had a teaching experience that most of them consider to be excellent. It's a shame *JAMA* didn't see fit to publish testimonials from any of them. . . .

Your publication of this piece suggests that unhappy experiences like Dr. Walker's are the rule at the Harvard Medical School; such is certainly not the case.

David C. Levin, M.D.

Editorial Note

It is beyond the ability of medical journals to ascertain the facts behind every opinion piece. As stated, we did not do so in the case of Dr. Walker's note, nor have we done it for Dr. Levin's response. We believe that readers looking at an article in a section headed ''A Piece of My Mind'' would not expect this. . . .

Our publication of Dr. Walker's piece does not suggest that Dr. Walker's experiences are the rule. Neither Dr. Walker nor, for that matter, Dr. Levin, produces any evidence bearing on this question. Among our editorial biases are these: that Harvard Medical School is a great institution but may not be perfect, that Dr. Levin loves it, and that, when there, Dr. Walker had a lousy time.

# CINÉ OR VÉRITÉ?

## Melanie S. Wayne, M.D.

Nine forty-five. I sighed, glancing at the clock in the emergency room. Typical, I thought, missing the only television program of the fall season that I really had wanted to see. The ironic injustice of it all! The patients who came to our clinic were so different from those I knew in my hometown or in the fancy big-city hospital at my medical school. I thought the documentary about sexually abused children might have helped this naive intern to know these kids when they showed up at our clinic. No such luck tonight, though—best to finish the paperwork now, so I could join the residents downstairs for a sandwich.

The triage nurse suddenly grabbed my arm, her face pale. I thought: "This woman makes it possible for the interns to survive the emergency department. If *she's* upset, it's a code. I know it. A code, and I don't know what to do. Is it five compressions and a breath, or . . . ?"

"Listen to me," she whispered shakily. "The police have a 10-year-old in the last room. She may have been raped. Please go talk to her," and her voice broke. When I saw the tears in her eyes, I remembered that she had a 9-year-old daughter at home.

Three burly police officers with notebooks and tape recorders were seated in the room, while a little girl huddled on the battered sofa across from them. Her dress was faded and frayed, and her dirty bare feet dangled above the grimy linoleum. Then I saw her face, tangles of hair partly hiding her wide, frightened face. She looked so small, so young, like a cornered animal afraid to fight. Her hands fidgeted in her lap, as she struggled to cover the stains in her dress and her dirty, broken nails. When we were alone at last, she said her name was Delores.

Delores told me what it was like to be abused by two men ever since the age of 5—whenever her mother left the house. She told me about wanting to run away, only to be too ashamed to tell the neighbors the real reason for leaving home. Then she begged me, with her tear-filled eyes burning holes in my heart, to keep her away from those men. I promised she would be safe with me tonight, and she gave me a little smile as she taught me the secret childhood handshake that made us "soul sisters."

After she was admitted to the children's ward, I took Delores upstairs to her bed. She clung to me until I promised to return in the morning, and when the sun came up I climbed the stairs again. My soul sister squealed with delight when I walked into her room, and she chattered animatedly about the cartoons on television, her delicious breakfast tray, the terrific house shoes the nurse had given her last night. While I gently brushed out her long brown hair, I wondered who loved this child. Was she really a child at home, or did she have to care for little brothers and sisters and babies in diapers?

Suddenly we were interrupted with news: Delores was going home! The two men were in jail and a social worker would take her home to her mother. I completed the paperwork, and she gave me one last bear hug and skipped down the hall in her disposable foam slippers, her shining brown hair sailing behind her.

Delores has not returned to the clinic or the emergency room since that night. I don't know what happened to the men who were arrested, or if she ever received any counseling through the city's department of social services. But I will never forget the night I cried in the call room, as if my own heart would break, the night I missed a television program and learned first-hand its valuable lessons.

# THE GUINEA FOWL

## Thomas E. Elkins, M.D.

Several years ago, at a "bush" hospital in rural West Africa, a small boy was brought by his worried parents to see the visiting American physician. The child had begun coughing and wheezing during the previous week. Now, his every breath required great effort and resulted in a loud, wheezing, grating sound. Asthma and pneumonia were diagnosed without any trouble, and every available medication (aminophylline, steroids, antibiotics, epinephrine,

B-agonists, intravenous fluid) was utilized. For five days, the 6-year-old child lay gasping with pleading eyes and whispered prayers. Nothing seemed to help, and oxygen and respirators were unknown in that part of the world. In a hospital where one nurse is responsible for 80 patients, IVs easily run dry at 2 AM. Even with a full hospital, the doctors come to the bedside two or three times each night to rewrite orders and to be sure that therapy is continuous.

On the fourth day of the hospitalization, the boy's father presented the American doctor with a prized possession as a gift: a plump guinea fowl. In a land racked by famine— where three onions could cost almost $30 in the market and a single pineapple fed a family for a week—a guinea fowl was a supreme sacrifice. The foreign doctor accepted the gift but was dismayed. The doctor's immediate concern was that this represented a "dash," or bribe, commonly required in parts of Africa to receive health care. He pulled an African nurse aside and asked if the father thought this "bribe" would make the physicians and nurses work harder and thus save the son, since the doctor was afraid the boy was going to die despite all efforts. The nurse looked hurt, and replied: "The father knows the son will die. He is grateful that you have tried so hard, and he wishes to share the guinea fowl in appreciation for the value you have placed on his son's life." The distrusting American physician felt ashamed and asked how he could share his gratitude with the father. The nurse suggested cooking the guinea fowl into a stew and sharing it with the family.

The next day, the physician and the family sat on the floor of the dimly lit, dusty children's ward and shared the stew. Even the small child, who was growing weaker, was able to eat some of the rich broth. Two days later, after all efforts had failed and the child was barely conscious, the family sadly carried him past the doctor, so that their child could die at home. There was no rush for an "against medical advice" form; no threats were voiced. The shared thankfulness had been fostered among physician, patient, and family—a covenant of understanding and, this time, a covenant also of sorrow.

Americans boast the greatest health care system in the world, while at the same time bemoaning a crisis in medical ethics, and an even greater crisis brought about by escalating malpractice litigation. In rural Africa, where the perinatal mortality approaches 15 to 20 per 100 births, where maternal death from uterine rupture is not rare, where "infection control" and "sterile environments" are misnomers, where supplies are severely limited, where hundreds of patients may try to see a single physician in one day, there are still insights to be gained by American physicians. Perhaps it is not too late for us to learn from the shared guinea fowl and covenant relationships in rural West Africa. As William May has implied, such lessons are based on the concept of "gifts" and an understanding of mutual gratitude.

# EQUAL, NOT REALLY

## Jane Marshall, M.D.

How can it be that at the age of 35, being an accomplished, respected physician, a happily married woman for 11 years, and a mother of two beautiful children, I feel melancholy, inadequate, and guilt-ridden? Ever since I can remember, my goals have been similar to those of most men. I have enjoyed competitive, physically demanding sports and achieved multiple varsity letters in high school. Excellence in general academics, and in particular science, was more important to me than even to my brother. The resultant conflicts of being a competitive and feminine woman in our society have been numerous. Nevertheless, I have always managed. In my 20s I was able to ride the early waves of "women's liberation." But now, at 35, the waves have crashed into the shore and eroded the sand.

My 6½-year-old gentle, vulnerable, and sensitive son has developed a "mild-to-moderate stutter." Stutter, stammer, and dysfluency are all different words for basically the same problem. My husband and I were recently called into our son's private school for a conference with his first-grade teacher, speech pathologist, director of the lower school, and assistant headmaster. During our hour together, we were informed that a probable causative factor in this was my working. Not enough mother-child time was the bottom line. It was strongly recommended that I alter my schedule if I felt "it was worth it." Worth it! Of course it was worth it!

Our initial response to this conference was anger. Both my husband and I were negatively impressed with our perception of these educators' lack of sensitivity to the plight of the "working mother" and "working couple." However, after serious review of our pressured and rushed life-style, I arranged an extended overdue vacation that corresponded with my son's school vacation. During this more relaxed intimate time together, his speech pattern became significantly more fluent. A partial solution to my child's stutter obviously included a more permanent change in my working schedule to increase our time together.

But what about my career and all the years of social deprivation to afford me more time to study? The years of "investing for my future" would now be set aside for something certainly more "worth it"! Worst of all there was my guilt. Why was I at fault? I have spent more time with my children than many nonworking mothers. My husband and I have almost completely eliminated our social and athletic activities in order to spend our free time with our children. This obviously was not enough for our more vulnerable eldest child!

I will, of course, alter my work load. I will curtail my teaching and publishing activities. I have a mind full of ideas that will not be written by me but by others.

Every time I hear my son speak, I feel his pain and frustration. I am filled with sorrow and guilt. I now know I am not equal to my male colleagues. In many ways I am better. However, I may not be allowed to show you or them because first I am a mother and wife and then I am a physician. I suppose I may continue to cry myself to sleep for many years. And when my daughter comes to me for career advice—what should I tell her?

*A good many people had answers for Dr. Marshall. Not surprisingly, most were other women physicians. Here is a sampling of the letters published in response to "Equal, Not Really."*

B. B. D.

To the Editor:

Every mother who works outside the home spends some moments feeling torn between the cradle and the work place and feeling guilty about the effects her outside work may have on her child. However, I must point out that there is no evidence that maternal employment has deleterious effects on children, although there *is* a lot of folklore out there. There is also no evidence that stuttering is caused by maternal employment. How cruel of the teacher, speech pathologist, and assorted administrators to state folklore as though it were fact! Sadly, this happens every day and physicians are often guilty. . . .

The woman *is* expected to care for the sick child, the aging parent, and the spouse. Although wives also fall ill, society views the husband's responsibilities toward illness in his spouse differently. The world is not yet helpful to, or even understanding of, the working mother. Yet more than half the women in this country with children are in the work force, most because they have to be there, not because they want to, as [the author] so desperately does.

I offer some advice to [the author]: (1) get another opinion on your child's stuttering, (2) consider another school, (3) join a group of parents of stutters, and (4) seek individual counseling. Don't let your anger toward the world, toward men who aren't expected to stay home, or even toward the child you love and want to help affect your decision, and (5) after carrying out suggestions 1 through 4, make your decision about working outside the home.

Marilyn Heins, M.D.

To the Editor:
Being grown-up means, among other things, knowing how to set realistic priorities, and this naturally involves making some sacrifices. . . . As the mother of two now fully grown, exceptionally sane, much loved children, I can look back on some years of severe financial disequilibrium, stress, and anxiety during our family's first decade. Throughout that period of unanticipated adversity, my husband and I *both* often felt "melancholy, inadequate, guilt-ridden," and desperate; certainly social and athletic activities never entered the picture. The difference between me and [the author] is that I had been dreaming of becoming a mother since age 8 or so, whereas she, apparently, has always invested her hopes in a distinguished medical career. The sacrifices I made came fairly easily—in fact, I enjoyed taking pains for my family—because these were consonant with my life goals.

Heidi Thains

To the Editor:
The fact that the final and often distant outcome of our choice can only be guessed at and cannot be known with certainty is an immutable fact of life. Trained surgeons have developed tremors and been forced to redirect themselves into second or third choices in medicine. Medical scientists have had to give up their research and go into clinical practice to support their families. Academic appointments have had to be refused or resigned because of unexpected conflicts with other priorities in a physician's or in his family's

life. The examples are endless, and every physician, male or female, has a personal disappointment or regret to add.

The "system" is not to blame for [the author's] present discontent, nor can the male sex take the blame. No one should take any blame. Hers is one of the contingencies of life that cannot be predicted. That the needs of a child may preclude experiencing the fullest measure of professional life was a definite possibility and would be known by anyone with the least experience in child development. She made her choice 7½ years ago when she became pregnant and should have realized then that life is not obliged to comply with anyone's wishes, however strongly they are held. Every physician, by having experienced his or her own personal disappointments, can understand the present disappointment of [the author]. No one, however, deserves the blame for life's uncertainties.

R. F. Sanke, M.D.

To the Editor:

I was most disturbed that this woman, her husband, and her son's teacher, speech pathologist, director of the school, and assistant headmaster all determined that the cause of her son's speech problem was because of *her* working. Why not because the child's father worked? She states that she will "of course" alter her work load. Why isn't her husband altering his?

I agree that this woman is not really equal because although she has a successful career in a demanding, male-dominated field and many attributes traditionally viewed as "masculine" (she is competitive and likes sports and science), she still believes that responsibility for her child's problems is hers alone. She will not be equal until she can realize that her son has two parents who are equally capable of "mothering" and demand that both parents do their share to help their troubled son.

As for what career advice to give her daughter, I hope

that her daughter doesn't ask for advice from a woman who has had so much guilt and pain from her own career.

Linda F. Ruekert, M.S.

To the Editor:
It is known that pediatricians often make judgments about maternal employment based on their own personal experience and biases rather than on scientific data. In fact, the majority of data reveal that there is no consistent effect of maternal employment per se on the intellectual or emotional development of children. Rather, outcome is determined by a complex interaction of such factors as the quality of substitute child care arrangements, family stability, parental attitudes toward maternal employment, and the quality of time spent with children.

Sophie J. Balk, M.D.

# CERTIFIED PINK

## Elliott B. Oppenheim, M.D.

The mailman became a hated figure to the physician on probation because he brought the certified mail with the familiar pink slip. "CERTIFIED" was written at least three times in red ink on each piece. As the doctor signed each succeeding pink slip, acknowledging receipt of these documents, he also acknowledged his crime and writhed in pain.

When his guilty plea appeared in the newspaper, two hospitals immediately terminated his privileges. Certified letters started arriving shortly thereafter.

When his license was revoked, certified mail announced the news. When the local medical society struck him from membership and two other hospitals removed him from the staff, more certified letters arrived.

His specialty organization hurled the next darts as his colleagues forced his resignation from the local, state, and national chapters.

The Drug Enforcement Administration next revoked his controlled substances certificate; another certified letter was on his doorstep.

Two more states revoked his license when they were notified by the federal government of the action involving his drug felony conviction; more certified letters, more pink cards.

His malpractice insurance carrier refused to renew coverage, and the doctor received a red envelope marked "URGENT, CONFIDENTIAL, CERTIFIED."

Loneliness and isolation had gotten him into using drugs initially, and now his colleagues abandoned and attacked him in his time of need. For all of his many years of medical practice, he now had a handful of pink cards to sign, each acknowledging failure, evidencing his conviction, and increasing his isolation.

As he handed him another certified envelope one day, the postman said, "You sure do get a lot of certified mail, Doctor. Say, are you practicing out of your home?" A patient who had read of his conviction lodged a complaint against him with the state Medical Disciplinary Board. The complaint lacked foundation, and the board never took any action, but they had investigated the complaint, and this added yet another pink card to his collection.

When a physician is convicted of a drug felony or in other ways transgresses accepted medical and social guidelines, resulting in license revocation or suspension, he must be punished and the public protected. But is there a way to lessen, somehow, the ostracism? If nominally maintained in medical organizations, even in a different category of membership, he would at least be eligible to receive mailings. He would then have a sense of belonging to something during his rehabilitation. Despite his misconduct, he is still a physician.

Does the physician's agony have to be compounded through termination of these career-long memberships? While I do not advocate continuing active membership in the medical society, the professional organization, the hospital staff, or even as a licensed physician pro forma, it seems hypocritical, and the antithesis of rehabilitation, to speak of rehabilitating the impaired physician on one hand and to banish him from the medical community on the other.

In a chilling study by Crawshaw et al., the State of Oregon Medical Disciplinary Board showed a shocking incidence of suicide in physicians on probation. There must be some way to keep a door open for our colleagues when so many doors have been slammed.

# NUMBERED BLESSINGS

## Neela K. Sheth, M.D.

It isn't easy to enter a hospice room and think of the right words to say. The cheerful "How are you today?" or "Hope you'll feel better tomorrow!" or "See you next week!" all carry loaded meanings and sound hollow, to both the "sayer" and the "listener."

My weekly visits as a volunteer started that Thursday evening with Helen, an elderly heavy-set woman with extensive bone metastases from a breast carcinoma treated many years ago. She lay on her bed slightly propped up, breathing heavily and moving her head monotonously from side to side. She alternately moaned and spoke in a soft, guttural tone as I walked to her side. I held her hand and began groping for some useful words to say. Then, gently stroking her hand, I tried to convey to her a nonverbal feeling that I cared about her. I slowly told her that I knew she wasn't well but that I wanted to be with her. After a few minutes, she seemed less agitated and more thoughtful. Then she began to cry softly, and through a hazy, muffled voice I thought I heard her whisper, "I want my mother."

Over and over she called for her mother, with tears streaming down her face. I continued to hold her hand and rubbed her forehead, listening, watching, sharing her pain and her remembrances of her childhood. Her confidence in me seemed to grow and I asked her about her mother. After much effort and in broken sentences she said that her mother lived in a nursing home in Iowa. The pain medications and Helen's somewhat confused state of mind made the nurse and me wonder if what she had said was indeed the current situation. So the nurse called Tom, Helen's husband, and told him that she thought Helen would be calmer and happier if she had a chance to see or at least talk with her mother.

Twenty minutes later I held the telephone to Helen's ear as she listened to Alice, her 91-year-old mother, on the other end. Helen's expression became intensely concentrated and she listened hard. She was responding to whatever Alice was saying to her, courageously answering, "I'm okay, Mama, but I miss you," "I love you too, Mama," and "Come soon, I'm waiting for Saturday."

All of this happened on Thursday evening. Helen was confused about hours and days and kept asking, "Oh, boy, when will it be Saturday, Tom?" and "How much longer do I have to wait?"

Alice flew in on Friday instead of Saturday; Tom must

have seen to that. It had been ten years since she had left the nursing home. I spent the week wondering about Alice and Helen and hoping they had a good visit.

I had lingering thoughts of Helen as I went back to the hospice the following Thursday. The log book showed Helen had died Saturday night. The nurse said it seemed a miracle that Alice in her severely crippled state could have even made the long trip to see her daughter.

Helen had willed herself to be with her mother before she ended her journey. She had waited for just that. As her life had begun 67 years before, it had ended now, in her mother's arms. She must have counted her numbered blessings . . . as must we all.

# THE WAITING ROOM

## Mark S. Litwin, M.D.

The intensive care unit (ICU) waiting room is a dismal place. Patients' relatives sit, waiting for the doctors to enter with hints of prognosis and wondering whether they are being candid or filtering out painful information. Families grope toward specific goals: "He'll recover; it's just a matter of time," or "She's dying; it would be better to get it over with."

Bernida, a 24-year-old mother, entered the ICU in status epilepticus. The corticosteroids she took for her lupus had been discontinued two weeks earlier, when she developed an acute psychosis. As her mental state improved, her disease flared, and she exhibited signs of lupus cerebritis. Late one evening, she began to have unremitting seizures. Intravenous tranquilizers did not quiet her, so she was transferred to the ICU, her body confused by abnormal signals from her ailing brain. But she was young and otherwise healthy, so the prognosis was good. Her mother, her husband, two brothers, and a sister moved into one corner of the waiting room.

Casey, an 84-year-old postman with chronic renal failure, entered the ICU in a stupor. Profound diarrhea and prolonged hypovolemia had thrown him into acute renal shutdown, and he was now receiving dialysis twice daily. His debilitated condition warranted admission to the ICU, his mind lethargic and confused by toxins in his sick blood. He was frail and ill, and his prognosis was poor. His elderly wife and their daughter claimed the other corner of the waiting room.

Every day after ICU rounds, the medical team made waiting room rounds. As we entered each morning, the room fell from chatter to silence. Hope-filled eyes firmly tracked our steps, as we moved in from the doorway.

Within a few days, both prognoses became clear. Bernida was recovering as expected. Although she waxed and waned, we chose to encourage her family's faith. With their confidence and positive attitude, Bernida would continue to get better. Casey, however, was deteriorating, and we decided to temper his family's optimism by gradually telling them some of the grim medical facts that led to our forecast.

Soon this became our daily agenda in the waiting room. Take away hope from Casey's family; build it up for Bernida's. The task was difficult, since each family overheard our comments to the crowd in the opposite corner. They did well at first, but after two weeks without change, Bernida's kin began to lose hope. And Casey's folks refused to surrender theirs.

The irony was frustrating, as our dual roles required more and more effort. Despite the patients' status, the waiting room took on a demeanor of its own. Hope leaked from one corner to the other, in the wrong direction. We tried earnestly to shift the flow, but the waiting room retained its strange backward balance.

One evening Bernida began to convulse again. The elusive etiology of her downward turn allowed us to treat her only symptomatically and blindly. The sudden shift from consciousness to spasm to barbiturate coma was too much for her family to accept, and they surrendered to the overwhelming stress. I implored them not to give up on her.

The next day, Casey's clouded consciousness began to clear. He resisted our predictions and showed signs of improvement. His abrupt change elicited delight from the fans in his corner, and they cheered as he seemed to regain his strength. I warned his family not to deceive themselves with unfounded optimism.

Patients sometimes unwitting defy their doctors. One day, we were surprised to find Casey sitting up and calmly reading a magazine. He had apparently dismissed his death. After confirming his stability, I rushed out to deliver the good news to his family. I swallowed my embarrassment for my previously tainted advice, as I shared in their relief. But I felt guilty: it wasn't my joy to share; I had condemned the man to death and was already preparing to ask for a postmortem examination.

I was equally perplexed that afternoon when Bernida died. After a tumultuous episode of seizures and metabolic complications, she dropped her natural defenses and fell to an unfair fate. Time ran out for her. As I walked to the waiting room, I felt like a naughty child who had just realized that his parents were right about something. I was ashamed to tell her family that she would not be coming home.

With deliberate optimism, Casey's family left the waiting room. They seemed relieved. With the same resignation, Bernida's family departed. They, too, seemed relieved.

I felt confused. Was I wrong to steal hope from one family and force it on another? Was my emotional Robin Hoodism inappropriate? I felt obligated to prepare these families for the inevitable, but my predictions were wrong. Only their own steadfastness saved them from my noble efforts.

As a physician, I command a powerful influence over people's hope. When there is none, I can often provide it; when there is too much, I can usually dash it. But isn't it hypocritical for me to deflate anyone's hope—even in the face of impending quietus? Perhaps I should leave odds-making for the bookies and uphold my responsibility to instill, not distill, hope.

I no longer believe that hope can be false. If it is all that a patient has, then who am I to take it away?

# THE BOARD CASE

## Lawrence M. Koplin, M.D.

I considered it a fortunate coincidence that he came to see me in the first place. I was in the infancy of my plastic surgery practice, at a time when any truly challenging patient is considered a windfall, an act of God, perhaps even a "board case."

Everett was 24 and handsome, with a large, deep malignant melanoma on his lower eyelid margin—a prognostic, anatomic, and cosmetic disaster. His understandably frantic mother took him from the dermatologist who had performed the original biopsy to another, perhaps in the hope of obtaining a better diagnosis. The dermatologist referred them both to a plastic surgeon, who was on his way out of town, and thus they were directed to me.

Everett seemed much less concerned than his mother or, as a matter of fact, than I about the seriousness of his problem. I presented everything as optimistically as I could.

They told me they had complete faith in my advice and ability, and I quickly put Everett on my rather uncluttered operative schedule.

I read everything I could lay my hands on. I talked with every plastic surgeon I knew. I dreamed—and awoke in the middle of the night—thinking about how to reconstruct the defect after I had excised the tumor. I had it all planned out, then changed my mind a hundred times. The day of surgery I was tense and anxious, waiting to begin but not absolutely confident of my plan or ability to execute it. Everett, in contrast, was relaxed, composed, smiling. I think his confidence, in part, helped the operation go as smoothly and successfully as it did.

Postoperatively, I barely slept for three days, waiting for the pathology report. I called Everett and his mother with the results—clear margins—from a pay phone at the Farmers Market on a Sunday morning. We were all thrilled and relieved when the bandages came off. Was I more surprised than Everett? At his one-month visit, he mentioned some irritation of the eye. An entropion had developed, with the lower-lid lashes rubbing the cornea. I was devastated. Everett was nonchalant; he knew I could correct it, and so I did. More sleepless nights. More agonizing. I finally settled on a cartilage graft from the ear and a little "plastic surgery" to the scars. My enthusiasm signaled a "great result," something that comes along rarely, that celebrates the best we have in us. I took a lot of photographs.

To achieve board certification, plastic surgeons must formally compile and present a series of cases they have treated since completing their residency. The cases must be drawn from nine diverse categories ranging from reconstruction of birth defects to major head and neck cancer surgery to cosmetic surgery. A board case is like the perfect wave to a surfer. It involves waiting, luck, and skill in varying combinations. Through the glow of having "rescued" Everett from possible death or disfigurement, I remember hearing an unconscious "click" as he fell into one of my required categories.

His mother telephoned about a month after the surgery to thank me. "He's back to normal, both physically and psychologically." I had tried to spend some time exploring Everett's emotional reaction to what I considered a stroke of incredibly bad luck. He seemed absolutely fine: cheerful, grateful, gracious. I was flattered that his mother had taken the time to call. I was riding the crest of a tall, azure wave.

Just three days ago his mother called again. Everett had been shot and killed the previous morning at the restaurant he managed, over a robbery of $200. He had been trying to protect a younger employee. As I sit here looking at his many pictures, my priorities come tumbling back into place. Yes, I am guilty of referring to him as my "melanoma case," and it is so easy to forget that every board case is a real person facing incredibly unfortunate circumstances with unimaginable bravery.

One of the great gifts of being a physician lies in the daily reminder of our own fragility, that the only difference between physician and patient is often, quite simply, "bad luck." Everett smiles in most of his photographs. His nonchalance reminded me of my own youthful disbelief in mortality, rekindling feelings of innocence and summers past that had not touched me since the beginning of my medical training—when *I* was 24.

I suppose I will be looking at Everett's picture one last time at my examinations this November, but I am not looking for any more board cases. I realize now that his mother had called me at the height of her grief to let me share it with her, because I had become a part of Everett's family for a brief moment in time. I know also that I received more from him than he had from me. Through his trust—total and unconditional—he helped me find the confidence to do a good job, to help me mature as both a surgeon and a person. There are no board cases. There are only people helping other people, one day at a time. Everett knew that. I only wish I could have thanked him for reminding me.

# After a Death

## Gregory S. Liptak, M.D.

I have witnessed many deaths and, loyal to my training, have generally remained objective and appropriately supportive during these events. Death, once a matter between family and physician, is now a public event involving guidelines, consultants, and tests, house officers, social workers, nurses, and students. This change in the nature of dying allows one to be more scientific and less involved when talking with a family, making it easier to review with them the litany of personnel and procedures that have been invoked and that basically mean there is no hope for their child.

I believe that, in general, I am too old to have new insights into myself; however, a death this summer became an epiphany for me. She was a 14-year-old girl, an only child, who three days earlier had been practicing to be a cheerleader, and who on a bright summer day, despite all our best skills and technology, had no life left in her brain. Her mother, a single parent, and her maternal grandmother sat by her bedside and waited for the end.

Her transition from life to death was quiet and private. The nurse and I closed the curtains around the bed; I wrote the order, showed it to the nurse, and turned off the power to the ventilator. The nurse disconnected the alarms, and we took up our stations on opposite sides of the room. While the mother held her child's head and the grandmother her hand, I watched them and the clock. For some reason tears started rolling down my face.

It is now considered acceptable for male professionals to cry at such times, as long as it is done noiselessly. Although I usually do not cry, I found myself crying for the life that had vanished, for the indescribable loneliness the mother would come to know, for the loss to the grandmother of a generation of women. I also cried for the child's regular physician, who had misdiagnosed the meningitis—was I so vulnerable too? But mostly I cried for my children, two healthy young boys. Like the Chinese who mourn the death of a baby when it is born, I mourned the death of my children while I watched this young girl die. I now carry part of their dying with me.

One of the most disconcerting aspects about disconnecting children from ventilators is that life often leaves with great reluctance. They shudder and gasp and twitch and inevitably lead you to believe that you have made a mistake and should not have disconnected them. She, however, was kind to us, and the rhythm of her beads and braids ebbed quietly.

We stayed in our positions, frozen like characters in an Edward Hopper painting, waiting. When the prescribed amount of time had elapsed for her death to be legal, I talked with the family and encouraged them to spend some time with her. They thanked me for everything we had done, although we had not really "done" anything to save her.

As I walked back to my office I thought about a friend, an obstetrician, who was being sued for the "wrongful life" of a child born with Down's syndrome. He had failed to send the 37-year-old pregnant woman for an amniocentesis. I wondered how life could be wrongful and considered that nothing in my childhood or education or training had prepared me to deal with such perplexities.

When I graduated from medical school I started a crusade to protect life from the dragon of death. Very gradually since then, death has become a fellow traveler—sometimes welcome, although usually not. I have vowed never to help him do his trade, yet I understand him a little more now and sometimes even converse with him.

Driving home, I thought about my children, who had picked raspberries for me the night before. My wife had told them that one of my favorite foods is fresh raspberries for breakfast. No food tastes as good, yet none is as perishable. I decided to stop at a local store to buy a whiffle ball and bat to thank them and to celebrate their living.

Our family lives in the country, surrounded by so many living things that death is a frequent visitor—especially to our canaries, who have been bred for song and beauty rather than for hardiness. We have a ritual: when a bird dies, we make it into a star. We troop outside to the boundary of our yard and throw the small body high into the air and into the adjoining wheat field. The body disappears in the tall grain before hitting the ground and makes no sound. That evening during supper we talked about the girl, and our 3-year-old asked if we had made her into a star. I told him we had and would point it out to him that night if he was still awake. I also told him I had placed a quarter in her hand when she had died in case she had to make a phone call; ''or play a video game,'' added our 5-year-old.

Friends often ask how I can do the work I do, especially the part dealing with death. I never know how to answer because I really do not know. Perhaps, like a gambler, I do it because I enjoy ''getting high on the action''; perhaps, like the hangman, I do it because it is a job that someone must do; or perhaps I do it from a sense of duty, borne out of my having been an altar boy and by hearing since childhood stories of family members who had been in the seminary. I thought I usually protected myself, however, by trying not to feel.

That night I dreamed that the girl's mother and I had taken her body to the edge of our yard and swung it back and forth. We heaved it toward the wheat field and like the canaries it disappeared in midflight with no sound. I sat upright, and then walked into our boys' room. I kissed each on the forehead and adjusted their covers. I wondered why

I did not feel more grief for this girl than I did, and I realized that I felt immense gratitude toward her. In her dying she was teaching me how to live.

# ONE COLD BEER

## Elizabeth Nolan, M.D., Ph.D.

Marie was a vivacious blond-haired, blue-eyed, 63-year-old woman. With her 70-year-old husband of 42 years, she worked hard to advance to a middle-class life-style. She had always been busily engaged in living, attested to by her starting college classes at age 60.

The diagnosis of sideroblastic anemia was also made at that time. It did not change her life-style, except to add the required transfusions to an already busy schedule.

When I first met Marie, I was a medical subintern picking up my next patient in the emergency department. Her family's chief complaint was that she was falling asleep all the time: Marie fell asleep in the middle of conversation, at the dining room table, and, tonight, while playing cards. Marie couldn't confirm or deny this because she was sleeping.

An extensive workup with numerous consultants at the university hospital revealed that Marie had hemochromatosis—the iron deposits from her frequent transfusions had infiltrated all parts of her body. It was as though Marie was full of rust. Indeed, the iron deposits prevented her heart from contracting effectively.

Physically, Marie needed a new heart; emotionally, hers

was the strongest heart ever. Marie loved and was loved by her extensive family.

Sometimes such families are difficult to manage. Marie's family was different. They waited attentively for the daily conference with me. They rationed their five-minute visitations. They were neat and clean, kept the children orderly, and wouldn't even bring a cup of coffee to the lounge. And they went home at night except for her husband and sons, who rotated the evening vigil so that Marie would always have someone there.

Their loved one had much to live for but little time left.

Now Marie was sleeping almost constantly. She asked frequently to see her husband and sons, who came readily only to find Marie asleep again.

The medications were failing her. Each day she needed higher doses and soon toxicities alone would compromise her body. Marie couldn't survive without these constant intravenous infusions and she couldn't live with the doses her heart demanded.

Although death is never certain, it is frequently expected. Patients and families unfamiliar with body functioning and medicines may not understand this the way medical personnel do. Patients and families look to other clues. To her loved ones, Marie was a beautiful woman resting peacefully. Her family was certain she would be going home soon.

But Marie would not be going home again. I told her husband and sons first, couching it in terms of her heart not being strong. I explained that her heart could pump effectively for a short period only. Then like a pair of tired legs, her heart had to rest for a while. The rest periods were increasing in frequency and length. Marie could never leave the intensive care unit.

I told her family that I was going to tell Marie. I felt she should know there might not be much time left.

I held Marie's hand, and began talking. Marie opened her eyes and smiled and then closed her eyes again. She held on to my hand and I knew she heard me say, "Be gentle with yourself, Marie, your family loves you." I told her that I didn't know what would happen or when, but that it was possible she could have a seizure or stroke or heart attack or that she just might not wake up from her sleep someday. I asked her what she would want us to do. Marie was very clear. She did not want to be intubated; she did not want to be on a ventilator. She said she was very grateful for all that we had done for her. She closed her eyes but held on tightly to my hand. And I held hers.

In a few moments, she opened her eyes and said, "Dr. Nolan, what am I supposed to do?"

Here was one gracious lady, knowing she was dying, that there was nothing modern medicine could do for her, and yet asking, "What am I supposed to do?"

I said, "Be gentle, Marie, there is nothing to do." I asked her if she had pain and she said no; I asked her if she was afraid and she said no; I asked her if there was anything that she wanted and she said no. Again she asked me, "What am I supposed to do?"

To myself I wondered, "What am I supposed to say?"

I told Marie to think about talking to her family. I told her they knew there was nothing to do. Marie released her hold on me and said, "Thank you, you are very kind." She said she would be OK and that she would figure out what she was supposed to do. "You can go now," she added. "I'll get you if I need anything." Then she fell asleep.

One half hour later I was paged to the ICU. I knew Marie wanted something. I hoped that we would be able to give it to her. She deserved whatever she wanted.

Marie was sitting up in her bed and appeared more strong than usual. I knew she seemed that way to me because of my own needs.

Before I could say anything Marie asked, "Dr. Nolan, would I be too brazen if I asked for a cold beer?" The simplicity of the request made me smile as I said, "Marie, you could never be too brazen."

I found Marie's husband in the waiting room and told him about her request.

"Too brazen?!" he exclaimed. "My Marie doesn't drink beer, she's never had a beer in her entire life!"

I said, "OK, that may be true, but if I were you I would get some cold beer and bring it to her. It's what she wants."

Marie had her cold beer, about 2 ounces. It was just enough to quench the thirsts of everyone who watched her smile.

When I left the hospital, Marie's family was still talking about that beer and I knew it was going to be a story many times retold.

Marie died that night. Many times I have told the story of Marie's first and last beer. It is a story of life and death, gentle and refreshing. And many times I have wondered, "What is it that we are supposed to do?"

# THE STATE OF THE ART

## Alvan R. Feinstein, M.D.

Her chief complaint is that she wants to die and that the doctors will not let her.

She is 96 years old. She has attended the burial of her husband, two daughters-in-law, and all the people who were close friends throughout her lifetime. A woman of fierce and independent spirit, she never wanted to live with her children, to be supported by them, or to be what she calls "a burden." After being widowed 24 years ago, she achieved those goals for a long time because she was in good health and her modest fiscal needs were met by the interest of the trust fund left by her husband.

Until 11 years ago, she lived alone and maintained her own apartment. She spent her time walking, talking with neighbors, reading, watching television, playing card games, attending religious services, and traveling to visit children, grandchildren, and great-grandchildren in different cities. At age 85, however, she began to dislike shopping and cooking for herself; and she began to worry about living 60 miles away from her nearest relative. She moved, in a city where a son and grandchildren lived, into an apartment residence building that was the "congregate setting" of a geriatric center. The setting provided her with lunch, dinner, a social life, and her own small apartment, in which she prepared her own breakfast.

On her 90th birthday, although in excellent mental and physical health, she began complaining that she had become too old. Her stated desire was to die in her sleep, preferably not on a night before she was scheduled to visit her great-grandchildren. When hospitalized with an episode of pneumonia that winter, she said, "My time has come." She bid a loving good-bye to each child, grandchild, and great-grandchild who came to see her, and gave them a farewell blessing. When she recovered—thanks to intravenous fluids and antibiotics—she was surprised and somewhat dismayed, but she resumed her former life, remaining independent and "perky."

During the next few years, she grew progressively more frail. She began having episodes of faintness, due to paroxysms of atrial fibrillation, but the episodes were brief, and the symptoms would vanish when she lay down briefly. She began walking with the aid of a cane. Although she would no longer travel long distances alone, her mind remained clear and her life independent. With each winter, however, she was rehospitalized with another bout of pneumonia. Each time she was sicker than before; each time she was prepared and wanted to die; and each time she received vigorous therapy and recovered.

During an episode three years ago, however, she had a spell of faintness while in the toilet of her hospital room.

Uncertain that she could successfully get back to her bed, she treated the symptom in her usual manner. She lay down calmly on the floor, closed her eyes, and waited. In that position, and with a rapid irregular pulse, she was found by a nurse, who promptly issued an emergency "Code" alarm. By the time the doctors and equipment arrived, she actually felt much better; but the excitement of the aggregated "team" convinced her she must be moribund. When she failed to die, she became angry and depressed. "I want to die, and I am ready to die," she said, "but the doctors won't let me."

After she returned to her small apartment, she became less depressed as she became persuaded that she needed to live at least another year to attend the religious confirmation of her youngest granddaughter. During that year, she became more frail, but her mind stayed clear and her spirits high. She traveled four hours in each direction by private car to go to the confirmation ceremony, and she took special pleasure in participating in it. During the trip, she laughed, sang, and joked, exchanging stories of the old days with a brother-in-law whom she seldom sees and who had come a long distance to ride with her to the ceremony.

Several days after her return home, she had a stroke. She became confused and disoriented. Although physically able to function, she could no longer take care of herself. She could not cook or successfully make her way alone to and from the dining room. When lucidity transiently drifted in, she would complain unhappily and bitterly about having a "companion," who had been hired to be with her during waking hours, and about having become "a burden."

About a week later, she re-entered the hospital with another, more severe stroke. She was conscious, seemed aware of her surroundings, and could state the names of her family visitors, but she made no other conversation. Moving her eyes toward the sky, she seemed to be pleading with God to take her at long last. When she developed anorexia, fever, and pneumonia, her children asked the house staff to let her alone, but they and the attending physicians insisted that they could not "do nothing." Before one of her sons—a physician at a medical school in a distant city—could arrive to dispute the doctors' plan, she was given intravenous antibiotics, fluids, and other vigorous support.

She recovered, left the hospital, and now resides in a nursing home. She can still recognize her family visitors, say their names, and engage in trivial conversation, but her mind is substantially destroyed. She does not know where she is or how long she has been there. She cannot read, watch television, walk alone, use a telephone, or play card games. She retains bladder and bowel continence, but she cannot dress herself, feed herself, or transfer from bed to chair to bathroom.

She is no longer aware of her plight, and expresses no suggestion of despair, but everything she wanted to avoid has happened. In a semivegetating state, she has lost her functional and mental independence; and she is about to become a financial as well as a physical burden. Because she has the trust fund, the government will not pay for the costs of the nursing home; but the trust-fund interest is not large enough to cover the charge of $80 a day. She had hoped to leave the trust-fund principal to her grandchildren, but now it will be gradually transferred to the nursing home.

As her visitors deal with the agony of her vegetation, they wonder why this problem has been created. Since the preservation of her life helps no one, and is desired neither by her nor by those who love her most dearly, why could her doctors not be content to let her die in peace and serenity? Why did they pursue a vigorous therapy that could benefit no one except their own satisfaction in thwarting death, regardless of the consequences?

I do not know the answers to these questions. But I, the physician son of this woman, weep for my mother and for what has happened to my profession.

# JOE

## R. Stephen Hillis, M.D.

One of my greater pleasures as a urologist is to converse with patients during operative procedures. Since many urologic procedures are performed under local or regional anesthesia, this opportunity comes often. I know that the anesthesiologist has in his arsenal a broad variety of sedatives to allay the anxiety inevitable with surgery, but an anesthesiologist is not always in attendance during procedures done under local anesthesia; even when there is an anesthesiologist in attendance, I inform him that I prefer to sedate my patients with my stories and resort to pharmaceuticals only when I do not get the anticipated relaxation. I have observed that the stress of a surgical procedure, however minor, and the unique relationship between surgeon and patient provide an environment for conversation that brings out emotions and philosophies heretofore suppressed by inhibitions. I know a patient better after half an hour in the operating room than after months of a more formal relationship.

Joe was a talker. I knew that long before he came to the operating room for transurethral prostatectomy. The preoperative medication did little to suppress this long-time habit. He talked constantly while in the holding area, talked while his gurney was wheeled to the operating room, talked as he moved over to the cystoscopy table, and continued to talk as the anesthesiologist and nurse held his chin to his chest and flexed his lumbar spine to facilitate entry of the spinal needle. I could practically read the mind of the anesthesiologist, who could not wait to get this chatterbox supine and slam home an intravenous bolus of his best sedative so that he could work in peace. Fond though I was of conversation, I began to agree that enough was enough.

After the injection into the subarachnoid space had been given, Joe was placed in the lithotomy position, and the chatter suddenly stopped. It was as though Joe's brain had been zapped by some pharmacologic cocktail, but in truth not enough time had elapsed to prepare and administer this. As it turned out, Joe's mind had been hit by a memory, and, as was his style, that memory lingered in his mind for only a few seconds before it found its way to his tongue and quickly filled the room.

Joe's memory took him to 1920, when he was 20 years old and was earning his livelihood as a pulpwood worker in east Texas. His 82-year-old body demonstrated muscle definition and tone that reflected the years of this physically demanding work. It was difficult, poorly compensated work that consumed most of a man's waking hours for most of the days of the year.

The day of which Joe spoke was a "day off" granted by his employer for a special reason. It seems that several months prior to this day, Joe had decided that life was rapidly escaping him and it was imperative that he begin to make some hard decisions, chief among which was to take a wife. As hard as this decision was, its implementation proved even more difficult. Rural east Texas was sparsely populated, and if one's work demanded one's waking hours for seven days every week, little time and energy remained for courtship. Joe resolved his dilemma by answering an ad found in the back of a magazine. The advertisement claimed that for a small fee one could obtain a list of proper young ladies who desired to marry but whose circumstances, like Joe's, were such that this desire was difficult to fulfill. Joe paid the required fee and as promised received the list of names with addresses and with a brief description of each young lady. Joe made his selection on the basis of geography, since his ability to travel was limited. It happened that one of the ladies lived just 25 miles away.

Joe was able to write and immediately did so, proposing marriage in his introductory letter (Joe had a habit of getting right to the point). The response came soon and was affirmative. So, Joe needed at least one day off to travel 25 miles by horse-drawn wagon, meet his bride, marry, return to his home, and set up house. Such a request seemed reasonable to his employer, who, along with the other workers, waited with an anxious curiosity to meet this "mail-order bride." Joe recalled that his employer warned him of swindlers who created schemes involving mail-order brides to rob a fellow of his life's savings. But Joe persevered on faith.

Joe returned home with a beautiful 16-year-old bride, anxious to flaunt his luck to his friends and fellow workers. Joe recalled that they all agreed that he had the prettiest wife of them all.

At this point in his narrative, Joe's chatter slowed down noticeably, enough that the work that had been going on as we listened with one ear came to a sudden stop. We anticipated that he either was completing a delightful story and was about to embark on another or was about to make a point and wanted the complete attention that he was receiving.

He held the pause long enough to pique our curiosity. We had known him long enough to wager that more was coming. His chin dropped to his chest and he spoke in a softer tone, staring as though looking through the ceiling. "We were married for 61 years," he said with a tone of seriousness and respect but with no noticeable remorse. No tears were evident on Joe's face, but a few began to appear on other faces in the room as we anticipated his next statement. After another brief pause he confirmed our suspicion: "I lost her last year." By now there were tears in many eyes, and the professional doctors and nurses, the supposed experts in comforting the distraught, looked at each other hoping that someone would know what to do, and would ease the grip of awkwardness by saying something trite or by offering a pat on the head while finally drawing a syringe full of something that would send Joe into a light, silent sleep.

Joe, however, stared at the ceiling for a few seconds, then cleared his throat. We realized the story was still not over and he had arrived only at the first plateau.

"Then . . ." he said softly and slowly. "Then . . . I got me a dawg." Tears suddenly dried and faces bore quizzical looks as we moved a little closer to hear what might come next. "Yep . . . I got me a dawg." Faces now tilted in looks of incredulity. "I loved that dawg so much," he said, his head moving side to side in a gesture of regret, "but I lost her, too . . . runned over on the highway."

"So . . ." We leaned forward in anticipation. "So . . . I told my kids . . . I said, 'You know, I'm lonely. I miss my wife and I miss my dawg. So when I get out of the hospital and get over this operation, I'm either gonna get me a wife or get me a dawg.' " A pin dropping would have been deafening. "So . . . when they brought me up here they told me, 'Daddy, when you come home we'll get you a dog.' So I am real anxious to get home."

Joe recovered and has done well. I have had the pleasure of seeing him at intervals, and I always inquire about his dog and I can hardly ask without holding back a little laugh and a little tear.

# DEATH BY MALPRACTICE

## Stanley Wohl, M.D.

It all began like so many other cases he had managed in his long career. The elderly patient had an incurable cancer, but required a minor surgical procedure to alleviate some troublesome symptoms. Everyone, including the patient, understood that the procedure was to be, at best, a palliative measure designed to make the patient's final few months a little more bearable. And he was a patient who remained as active as possible and who clung to life with all his might. He was blessed with a caring, loving family whose members were unanimous in requesting that the procedure be done. The tumor board recommended it. It was to be routine.

The surgeon took on the case as a favor to a colleague. He certainly did not need the work. At 63, he was trying to curtail his busy operating schedule. For 30 years he had been the busiest general surgeon in town. He was fast and he was good and, as a consequence, physicians and their families constituted a significant proportion of his practice. His children were educated and married. The last thing he really needed at the time was another Medicare case. But the case was referred to him by a colleague and friend and he always had trouble saying no.

There are those cases, and we all know them well, that seem to go downhill from day one, regardless of our best efforts. There is seldom a reason. They just don't work. All busy physicians have experienced the frustration involved in the management of such a case. The best brains and hands in medicine, using state-of-the-art technology, sometimes produce poor results. And it can happen in the most routine of clinical situations, as if Mother Nature were just waiting for us on that particular day. When it does occur, one is reminded of the fact that patients are not machines and that they sometimes react to appropriate, competent therapy in unexpected ways.

This was, unfortunately, one of those cases. The trouble began with the administration of the anesthetic and then, for one postoperative week, things went from bad to worse, until the unfortunate patient died. It was a textbook case of the physician's theory on nightmares: in health care, whatever can go wrong sometimes does. Almost every medication prescribed induced an allergic reaction. Precipitates formed in clear intravenous solutions. Every vein touched by a needle thrombosed. Catheters got blocked. And late one night, the light above the patient's bed simply exploded and showered the room with glass.

Through it all, the family seemed to understand and in the end expressed their gratitude for the efforts made. The referring physician had maintained his close relationship with the family throughout the difficult postoperative week. The surgeon developed an excellent rapport with the family and, as was his style, was completely honest, available, and forthcoming with detailed information during the week. Even during some of the roughest moments, the family never once expressed dissatisfaction with the care that was provided by the nursing and orderly staff. Almost everyone involved in the patient's care received a warm letter of thanks two weeks after the patient's death.

The lawyer's letters, however, began to arrive four months later. The family had unexpectedly decided to sue the surgeon and the hospital in a personal damage action on behalf of the patient's estate. There followed another year of subpoenas of records, depositions, wrangling with insurers over settlements, and heated exchanges among the multitude of interested parties because the surgeon did not wish to settle out of court. The patient's death continued to haunt him because he could not explain it, but being accused of inflicting damages—death, in this case—was not an issue he was prepared to leave uncontested. Despite his carrier's decision to abandon him because he refused to settle out of court, and despite the hospital's decision to revoke his privileges because he was now "bare," he awaited his day in court.

He waited for two years. But while he was waiting and waiting, his appetite waned and he lost considerable weight. He had trouble sleeping, and his wife of 40 years found him almost unbearable to live with. Colleagues and friends tried to break through the curtain of depression, but to no avail. The finest attorneys in the country assured him repeatedly that no jury would find him responsible for that patient's unfortunate death. But it all ended in a hotel room with a bottle of pills and a note of apology. He never did get his day in court. He just could not wait that long.

There undoubtedly were other problems troubling the surgeon, but neither his wife nor friends could determine what they were. Advancing age, impending retirement, and the "empty nest syndrome" probably played their part in the depression, but the malpractice problem, coming as it did so late in a magnificent career, was the elbow that pushed him over the edge. It was the surgeon's first and only accusation of malpractice, but it was fatal. For whatever reason or combination of reasons, he simply could not deal with it in a realistic manner.

There are those who claim that the primary cause of the current malpractice dilemma is malpractice itself. Others point the finger at a litigious society bent on abusing the tort system for personal gain. Irrespective of the merits of the differing points of view or of the merits of the actual lawsuits initiated, it would seem reasonable for all parties to work toward reforms that would speed these cases into a court of law. It is in the waiting for judgment that careers and lives are destroyed.

# Rites of Passage

## Charles W. Jarvis, M.D.

The rituals of retirement had come to an end. The hospital tea had come first. It was much like all the many, many retirement teas I had attended over the decades. People from all walks of life and all areas of the hospital had stood in line to wish the honored one well, to share a new joke, to ask about plans, and then had gathered in little talking knots about the long tea table. The table, as usual, was resplendent in white linen, the best tea service, tiny sandwiches, salted nuts, the regulation garlic-flavored cheese ball, and, at each end, an attractively dressed pourer (tea or coffee?) from the department. The administrator had made a gracious speech to light and polite clapping from the assembled group. Yes, it had been a mirror image of a thousand other farewell teas, only this time I was at the wrong end of the line, the attractively dressed pourers were from my own department, and the administrator was talking about me. After the hospital tea came the lab party, a glorious time of goodwill where I finally was permitted to kiss each of the beauties I had hired over the years. The medical staff dinner had come last in the guise of a "roast" at which I might have cried, had we not all been too busy laughing and eating to have room for tears.

The files in the office had been easy to clean out, and in the end only a few things went home. In the den the debris and the detritus accumulated in 30 years were not as easy to discard. The microscope, in an unfamiliar new plastic jacket, went on a shelf by my desk—spring and growing grandchildren might yet find delights in the pond behind the house with its help. Unread journals (how old?) were gradually weeded out with only a minimal number of articles saved. (For what reason? Lo, the habits and enthusiasms of a long love affair with medicine.) There were a few rejected manuscripts of my own to reread (yes, they should have been rejected) and a number of textbooks that were both too new and too old to be worth keeping. There were also the printed cullings of innumerable educational meetings— local, state, and national—that finally had to give way to progress.

As the weeks went by there seemed to be a core of things that kept being saved miraculously from the trash. There was the freshman gross anatomy book (that subject doesn't change, just the presentation), a series of color transparencies of diseased organs (rather good quality, but where can one find a projector that will handle $2\frac{1}{4} \times 3\frac{1}{4}$-in lantern slides?), a folder containing bizarre electrophoretic patterns (paper electrophoresis, even yet?), a sizable collection of photomicrographs of cells, some beautiful, some only bizarre (sperm in gastric washings of a premature infant?), even a telephone list-finder that traced the changing pattern of my referrals over the decades.

For some reason, these and other items didn't throw away easily. At first I didn't notice the tiny pang that occurred each time I viewed these items, which seemed to have developed lives of their own. Then one day I discovered a small group of color slides that made me realize what was happening. These slides from many years ago were of people. There were only four people at first, all young, all handsome, all smiling, and all working in a tiny, primitive lab. With the sight of them came a flood of memories— memories of how we set up the first paper electrophoresis system in town, of how we taught ourselves to make our own agar gel strips and our own iontophoresis equipment to induce sweating. There were memories of our first case of leukemia (a boy, age 3) and how inexorably fast he died, of our first flame photometer and our first pH meter for blood, and of how we struggled to develop anaerobic methods for obtaining capillary blood. There were memories of new procedures, of new equipment and new personnel, of medical technology students we taught together, and of our constant drive to unlearn old falsehoods.

I sat back and wallowed in the emotions that the pictures brought out—poignant, humorous, and sad. After a while I began to feel guilty; grieving for my lost youth, was I, now that the years seemed to have shoved me aside? Perhaps. Perhaps not. Youth seems to be full of excitement, of course, but it's really life that's full of excitement, life and change, not just youth. The excitement had been from within and represented our own growth.

The telephone rang. It was from one of the beauties in the old photograph—still as lovely as she had been when the slide was taken. She wanted to tell me about a person she had met recently, a former patient we had worked for together, who now had children of her own. "Remember," she said, "she was a newborn who had erythroblastosis and we couldn't crossmatch her with Rh-negative blood because she was sensitized to little c. It was the first case of its type we'd ever seen, and we solved it together." No, the excitement hadn't come from our youth, it had come from challenges met and overcome, usually together. Suddenly I knew that the artifacts on my desk could now be discarded, all except the pictures of people. I had completed another passage, not come to an ending.

I put the phone down and swung my chair around to face the table behind me, thinking of the future. How many stories there were to tell. I threw a switch and slipped a thin disk into the base of the computer sitting there. When the screen cleared, I selected 10-point Geneva, plain text, six lines per inch, double spaced, and started to type:

### NIGHT WATCH

The night supervisor's voice on the telephone said, "Lab?

Can you bring your tray right over to ER? We have a very sick newborn here with deep jaundice and . . .''

Rites of passage belong not just to the young, but to all ages, even unto retirement and beyond.

# LAST IMPRESSIONS

## Lawrence M. Linett, M.D.

I disliked him immediately.

He was one of the last patients I worked up during my internship, a seemingly interminable year that was finally coming to a close. His diagnosis was inoperable lung cancer, the deadly seed of which had already blossomed in his liver and bones. He had refused chemotherapy in the past, consenting only to local radiation therapy. Concerned about his increasing confusion, hostility, and disorientation, his family had brought him that night to the emergency room for evaluation.

As I approached him, I could sense his hostility. He looked older than his 72 years; the ravages of cancer were obvious in his pasty complexion and marked muscle wasting. His eyes sat deep in their sockets, and the sparse white tufts of hair on his head reminded me of dead trees on a mountain ridge.

"I don't like doctors and I don't want to stay," he began. "Who are you anyway? You'd better not be a medical student! The last time, a student tried for an hour just to get some blood from me!" I assured him that I was indeed a licensed M.D., being careful not to bring up the gulf between my experience and that of a staff physician. With some reluctance he let me draw blood and examine him. I found nothing significant other than a few "crackles" at the lung bases and a moderately enlarged and tender liver. He was certainly oriented to time and place, but his anger and combativeness were still sufficient to show why he had been brought in. The emergency room is always open, a fact that is of great relief to tired and frustrated families.

I suspected metastasis to the brain, and I began to explain the need to admit him for a CT scan. He immediately became indignant. "Why you little bastard, I don't need to stay here. You doctors are all worthless. As for you, you barely look old enough to be in college!" At 3:30 in the morning, I was in no mood to argue. His family tried, and he remained hostile and combative but finally agreed to stay.

His mood was no better the next morning. One of the nurses said jokingly that she would take the rest of the week off if assigned to care for him again.

When his cranial CT scan showed no sign of malignant spread, I decided to look for emotional or psychological reasons for his hostility. With trepidation I approached his bed, sat down beside him, and asked, "Would you mind telling me a bit more about what you've got wrong with you?" He said he knew he had metastatic lung cancer, that it was going to kill him, and that he was willing to accept his fate; it was his family that kept bringing him for evaluation "at the drop of a hat."

"Makes you sort of mad, doesn't it?"

"I just want to die at home," he said. "Save your fancy technology for someone else. I don't want your tubes and catheters; I want to go while *I'm* still in charge of my life."

When I admitted that tubes and catheters wouldn't help him get well, he relaxed and much of his hostility disappeared.

"When I first found out I had cancer," he said, "I denied it, like anyone would. Then I became angry—with my family, my friends, my doctor; I blamed them all for what was happening to me." He paused for a moment, staring into space. "I was mad as hell, too," he continued, "because they were all telling me what to do. *I* was the one with the cancer; *they* were the ones making the decisions. I read up on cancer and talked with people who had had chemotherapy. I decided I had lived a good life and the doctors could keep their chemotherapy and its side effects. I had done all I wanted to do in this world and it was time to leave it my way."

A certain belligerent set came back to his jaw, and he said, "I can honestly say I'm at peace with myself and my decision. Tell my family that," he said, tapping my chest with his finger. "Tell them there's nothing you can do—and nothing I would let you do even if you could!"

We spoke for a while longer about cancer and the ways it affects a person and his family. He mentioned friends who had died of cancer and the pain some had had. "That scares me," he said, looking away from me. "I'm in pain most of the time now, but I was brought up not to show suffering—to be stoic. Lord knows if my family learns about the pain, they'll hover over me like I'm a helpless baby. I know I'm giving them a hard time, but fighting is all I have left—all I have to remind them that I'm still capable of running my life." I asked if he could talk about all this with his family, and he said, "No, it's my problem, and I'm going to stay in control."

I admired his courage, and I wondered if I would be as brave in the same situation. I learned more about the complexities of cancer from him than from any textbook I had read. And when I left him that day, I found that my hostility, like his, had disappeared.

I had mixed emotions when he was discharged the next morning. He had his wish to go home. For that I was glad and I hoped he wouldn't have to come back, but I knew I would miss a man I had come to like.

# IN THE BACK OF THE AMBULANCE

## Robert Marion, M.D.

I was scheduled to be the Early Bird and so, after trudging sleepily through the cold, predawn morning, I entered the pediatric emergency room just before 6 o'clock. It was the third month of my internship. I was exhausted and felt as if I'd had enough. Jeff Goodman was sitting in an examining booth, finishing off a chart. "How was your night?" I asked, sitting next to him.

"If I live to be a hundred," Jeff answered, "I'll never understand why people bring kids to the ER at 5 AM for diaper rashes." He finished the chart and said, "Look, it's quiet. I'm going to take a nap in the isolation room, okay?"

"Sure," I said nervously. "You mind if I wake you up if I have a problem?"

"I expect you to wake me up if you have a problem," he answered. "You know where to find me." And he shuffled off toward the back of the ER.

I was praying no patients would show up before 9 o'clock, the time when the rest of the staff arrived, but my hopes were dashed when a 6-year-old boy who had been bitten by a German shepherd checked in 45 minutes later. I carefully examined the child's wrist, which bore some scratches and a puncture hole. Not even having a clue as to what to do, I began heading for the isolation room. Lynn, the ER's head nurse, intercepted me. "Where do you think you're headed, pal?"

161

"The isolation room," I answered, "to wake up Jeff."

"You're planning to wake up Jeff for a dog bite?" she asked.

"He told me to get him if I needed help," I answered.

"Look, you need help with a dog bite, you ask me, okay? A kid with meningitis comes in, you can wake up the resident. Understand?"

Intimidated, I nodded and meekly asked, "Well, what should I do?"

"You check to see if the kid's had a tetanus shot recently, you give him a seven-day course of penicillin, and you tell him to stay away from that dog. What the hell's a kid doing getting bitten by a dog at 6 in the morning, anyway?"

I didn't answer but turned back to the boy and his mother, who had heard this interchange, and did exactly as Lynn had instructed. They departed at 7:30, and on the way out, the mother stopped to thank Lynn for her help.

I was beginning to relax when the paramedics came in at 8 o'clock. "Morning, Lynn," I heard the brown-haired one say. "How's business?"

"Fine until you guys showed up," she replied. "What bundle of joy do you have for us this morning?"

"We've got a SIDS in the back of our wagon," the red-haired guy said. "A SIDS?" Lynn asked, panicking. "You think you might want to bring the kid in so we can do some resuscitation?"

"Not on this one," the brown-haired paramedic said slowly. "The mother found her cold and stiff a little while ago. Pupils were fixed and dilated when we got there and the corneas were clouded over."

"We don't even want to bring her in," the red-haired guy added. "All we need is a doc to declare her, and we'll haul her down to the morgue."

I rose and started again for the isolation room, but Lynn caught my movement out of the corner of her eye and yelled, "Bob, get over here!"

"Don't you think Jeff oughta take this one?" I pleaded,

obeying Lynn's command and edging slowly toward the group. "I don't even know what to do."

"There's nothing to it," Lynn said. "You just go out there, make sure there's no heartbeat, and say she's dead. It's no big deal."

"What about the parents?" I asked. "What do I tell them?"

"No problem," the brown-haired man said. "They're coming on their own." "Move it, Bob," Lynn ordered, "before we start getting backed up."

Complying with her order, I nervously followed the paramedics out into the ambulance port. I hadn't yet been alone with a dead human being. Although I had seen and touched the dead in medical school, I had always been accompanied by another student or an intern. Now I was the intern, and I was alone. My flesh began to crawl.

She was lying on a stretcher in the back of the cold ambulance. She was covered with a blanket, but I could make out the bulge that was her head, the one that was her trunk, the ones that were her legs. Goose bumps popped up on my skin; my impulse was to run, but when I turned and eased out of the ambulance, the paramedics were waiting there for me. "All you have to do is say the word and we'll cart her down to the morgue," the red-haired one said.

Unable to run, I softly said, "She's . . . she's dead."

"You can't declare her unless you see her," the brown-haired one whispered.

My legs began to feel wobbly, but I walked back into the ambulance and began slowly to lower that blanket. First her brown hair was visible, then her eyes, then slowly her nose and mouth, and finally there was the whole face.

She was beautiful, with fine, doll-like features. "She's 4 months old," one of the paramedics said, his voice breaking the icy silence.

Looking at her, I had trouble convincing myself she was actually dead. I pulled the blanket down suddenly, exposing the chest, and whipped out my stethoscope. I listened hard, concentrating on trying to hear heart sounds. "She's got a rate," I finally said in a panic. "It's beating about 120 times a minute."

"Bull!" the red-haired paramedic said, tearing the stethoscope from my ears and putting the earpieces into his. "There's no heartbeat, Doc. You must be hearing your own heart."

I put the stethoscope back into my ears and realized he was right. "She is dead," I sighed. Quickly, the paramedics covered the body and prepared to drive off.

It was then that the tears began to come. As I stepped out of the back of the ambulance, I tried to stop them but couldn't. I realized I was crying not only for this child, but for myself. I had spent four years in medical school, had lost sleep at night studying, thinking this would prepare me to be a good doctor. Now I was a doctor, and it was on this morning that I finally had to admit to myself what I had known since the day I had started my internship: that I was inadequate, that my training had not prepared me to help people, that I couldn't even treat trivial problems like dog bites, that I was throwing away the best years of my life trying to work toward a goal seemingly as impossible to reach as trying to bring that baby in the ambulance back from the dead.

After a few minutes, Lynn came out to find me. "Move it, pal," she said, "this isn't rest period," but then, seeing the state I was in, she put her hand on my shoulder and led me back into the ER.

Inside, Jeff was seeing a patient. Lynn led me into the isolation room and called Jeff over stat. The resident left his patient and, muttering, "This had better be important," entered. He took one look at me sitting on a chair, holding my head in my hands, sobbing softly, and asked, "What happened, Bob?"

When I couldn't answer, Lynn said, "I sent him out to declare a SIDS and I found him like this in the ambulance port."

"Your first dead baby?" Jeff asked. I nodded. "I remember mine," he continued, flopping down on the room's other chair. "A kid who fell out a fifth-story window. He barely had a scratch on him. No problem at all except he was dead. I felt pretty helpless. I had nightmares about it for months."

I had calmed down a little by that point. Jeff and Lynn stayed with me until they were called out: a 10-year-old had been brought in in the midst of a long convulsion. I remained in the isolation room for two hours. At 10:30, I stepped into an ER buzzing with activity and filled with residents, medical students, and patients, and I began to pick up where I had left off.

# THREE FEET TALL
# AND THIRTY POUNDS

## Michael R. Clemmens, M.D.

We met late one night in the pediatric intensive care unit. He was the patient; I was the intern. Earlier that day he had been exploring his world with a vigor that only a 3-year-old could know. He had found a parked motorcycle, tried to climb aboard, and succeeded only in pulling it over, pinning himself beneath it. He was found moments later, nearly lifeless. The wonders of basic and advanced life support restored his heartbeat, but he was still in a deep coma when he arrived in the ICU that night.

At first glance he seemed the prototypic 3-year-old: three feet tall and thirty pounds. He was just beginning to lose his toddler's potbelly. Blond and fair-skinned, he had blue eyes that hours before must surely have twinkled with warmth and excitement. But now they were glazed, his stare empty and searching. His brain had begun to swell, unwilling to forgive him his breathless moments.

How he captured my heart is not at all clear to me now. Perhaps he conjured up feelings attached to some other little boy I had once known but whose name and face I had long since forgotten. Perhaps he resembled too closely my vision of a child I hope someday to father. Or perhaps he and I merely happened to meet at a time when we were both particularly vulnerable, he physically and I emotionally. In whatever mysterious way it happened, the bond was formed. Of all the patients I had cared for in my brief career, he seemed to matter the most. Pascal said, ''The heart has its reasons which reason does not understand.''

But after several days of heroic medical efforts the swelling in his head continued to progress. It became clear that his brain was no longer accepting blood flow from his heart. When the ''life'' support systems were withdrawn, the completion of his death came quickly.

Although I stayed with the family during those final hours, my tears refused to flow. It was only later, alone in the on-call room, that I embraced the pain of the loss that was still such a mystery to me.

The following day was St. Patrick's Day, and I sat watching the parade from the curb, alone in the midst of the crowd. There was the usual procession of bands and floats, and then a little boy, blond, blue-eyed, about three feet tall and thirty pounds. He looked me straight in the eye and asked, ''Can I sit on your lap to see the parade?'' Together we watched and clapped and laughed and cheered.

"It's Over, Debbie" was certainly the most controversial "A Piece of My Mind" and perhaps the most controversial article ever published in JAMA. Its publication stirred up a furor in the medical community, the press, the legal fraternity, and the lay public. The article dealt with the taking of a life by a physician, whose name was withheld by request. "Debbie" became the subject of dozens of newspaper, radio, and television stories. It was the center of attention on a "Good Morning America" segment featuring medical, legal, and media experts.

"Debbie" was no less controversial among The Journal's own staff. Several of the editors objected to it, stating that its publication was inappropriate and potentially harmful. JAMA's editor, Dr. George D. Lundberg, later stated in numerous interviews that he wished to publish it to stir the debate about euthanasia, but many medical ethicists said that this was not a case of euthanasia—it was murder. In fact, in response to media pressure, the Illinois State Attorney's office issued a subpoena to obtain the name of the physician who submitted the article.

For those who have never actually read the now infamous essay, here it is in its entirety, along with a series of just a few of the letters that JAMA received after its publication. Of interest is that, of the hundreds of letters from physicians, most objected to the article's publication and condemned the action of the doctor in question. Of the hundreds received from the lay public, most commended the doctor for having the courage to relieve a patient's suffering. Read it and make your own decision.

# IT'S OVER, DEBBIE

## Name Withheld by Request

The call came in the middle of the night. As a gynecology resident rotating through a large private hospital, I had come to detest telephone calls, because invariably I would be up for several hours and would not feel good the next day. However, duty called, so I answered the phone. A nurse informed me that a patient was having difficulty getting rest, could I please see her. She was on 3 North. That was the gynecologic-oncology unit, not my usual duty station. As I trudged along, bumping sleepily against walls and corners and not believing I was up again, I tried to imagine what I might find at the end of my walk. Maybe an elderly woman with an anxiety reaction, or perhaps something particularly horrible.

I grabbed the chart from the nurses' station on my way to the patient's room, and the nurse gave me some hurried details: a 20-year-old girl named Debbie was dying of ovarian cancer. She was having unrelenting vomiting apparently as the result of an alcohol drip administered for sedation. Hmmm, I thought. Very sad. As I approached the room I could hear loud, labored breathing. I entered and saw an emaciated, dark-haired woman who appeared much older than 20. She was receiving nasal oxygen, had an IV, and was sitting in bed suffering from what was obviously severe air hunger. The chart noted her weight at 80 pounds. A second woman, also dark-haired but of middle age, stood at her right, holding her hand. Both looked up as I entered.

The room seemed filled with the patient's desperate effort to survive. Her eyes were hollow, and she had suprasternal and intercostal retractions with her rapid inspirations. She had not eaten or slept in two days. She had not responded to chemotherapy and was being given supportive care only. It was a gallows scene, a cruel mockery of her youth and unfulfilled potential. Her only words to me were, ''Let's get this over with.''

I retreated with my thoughts to the nurses' station. The patient was tired and needed rest. I could not give her health, but I could give her rest. I asked the nurse to draw 20 mg of morphine sulfate into a syringe. Enough, I thought, to do the job. I took the syringe into the room and told the two women I was going to give Debbie something that would let her rest and to say good-bye. Debbie looked at the syringe, then laid her head on the pillow with her eyes open, watching what was left of the world. I injected the morphine intravenously and watched to see if my calculations on its effects would be correct. Within seconds her breathing slowed to a normal rate, her eyes closed, and her features softened as she seemed restful at last. The older woman stroked the hair of the now-sleeping patient. I waited for the inevitable next effect of depressing the respiratory drive. With clocklike certainty, within four minutes the breathing rate slowed even more, then became irregular, then ceased. The dark-haired woman stood erect and seemed relieved.

It's over, Debbie.

To the Editor:

Has briefly prolonging life in doomed patients taken priority over providing for their comfort? Are our technologically oriented hospital physicians as unfeeling as our proliferating critics say we are? Does it take a formal hospice program for this kind of patient to receive appropriate care (I hope not)? Hospital staffs or attending physicians who allow a terminal patient to suffer like this patient should be spotlighted by name, not protected. . . .

Physicians of all specialties and levels of training who

see dying patients in pain and distressed patients deprived of adequate comfort despite "supportive" or "keep comfortable" orders should speak up: They should not, sneakily and in the middle of the night, dispatch the patient, as if attaining a pain-free state were not a respectable, attainable, primary goal.

Bernadine Z. Paulshock, M.D.

To the Editor:
I was distressed by the article . . . "It's Over, Debbie." I, too, was a tired gynecologic resident rotating through large hospitals and I saw similar situations and, perhaps, responded no better than our nameless physician. . . .

I have learned that patients like Debbie do not need to be killed by their physicians to be relieved of their shortness of breath. . . .

Porter Storey, M.D.

To the Editor:
"It's Over, Debbie" constitutes a textbook example of medical arrogance, ignorance, and criminal conduct. We plan to use it as a teaching vehicle in courses at our medical school, law school, and school of public health. Truth can indeed be more frightening than fiction. Thank you, Debbie, for reminding us.

Frances H. Miller, JD
George J. Annas, JD, MPH

To the Editor:
I was deeply impressed by the article entitled "It's Over, Debbie." I would like to extend my most enthusiastic congratulations to the author for having the courage to submit this account.

Faced with a similar situation as a resident some years ago, the morphine approach seemed to be the obvious solution. But I just didn't have the strength to relieve a young man's suffering in view of the possible repercussions of such an action. It is encouraging to learn that at least one of us has risked his career to relieve the suffering of another.

Charles B. Clark, M.D.

To the Editor:
I am outraged by the action of the physician in this case who served as jury, judge, and executioner of this young patient, and I believe that the vast majority of physicians feel the same way. I also strongly protest *JAMA*'s publication of this article. It casts the medical profession in a very unfavorable light. Is it any wonder that most polls in recent years have shown that physicians are not held in as high esteem as they used to be?

John G. Manesis, M.D.

To the Editor:
If the physician who helped Debbie to die had acted as he did in Holland now, or in America in the future when the Humane and Dignified Death Act is passed, he would be prosecuted.

Dutch rules, and the proposed act in the United States, are clear that a request to be helped to die must be in writing and must have been carefully considered. Also, *two* physicians must agree that the patient is dying. The family must be informed but cannot veto the patient's wishes.

You have done a service to both the medical profession and patients by publishing this essay and demonstrating in at least one instance how poorly hospitals handle such requests for euthanasia.

Incidentally, 20 mg of morphine is not likely to be a fatal dose. My guess is that it put the poor young woman into a sleep, during which she died. That was compassion.

Derek Humphry

To the Editor:
Debbie's life is over. Also, over, however, is the tenet that killing is an act that our society finds abhorrent. That the resident could kill a patient, let alone one whom he did not know or with whom he had no relationship, represents a breach of any semblance of medical ethics and the rule of law. That *JAMA* could publish this cavalier description of homicide, however, bespeaks a social milieu that is tolerant to the killing of patients by physicians.

Over is an era when the physician's goal is to restore the health and well-being of the patient or, if he cannot achieve this, to withhold or withdraw life-sustaining therapies and provide adequate analgesia, care, and company to relieve the suffering and despair of the patient. The ancient medical dictum of "to cure sometimes, to comfort always" has become "to cure sometimes, otherwise to kill." . . .

Over is the ethic of the caring physician. Instead, we see emerging the ethic of the killing physician. Over is the ethic of the helping profession. Instead, we see emerging the ethic of the killing profession. If any one physician kills, the mission of our entire profession is endangered. Our civilization had an experience with systematic and institutionalized medical killing earlier in the century; many of us naively thought this experience was permanently behind us. Apparently, the killing of patients by physicians is no longer inconceivable to the medical public or American society. It's not over, Debbie, it's only just beginning—again.

Peter A. Singer, M.D.


To the Editor:
I am sure there are a lot of my colleagues who may be shocked by the article entitled "It's Over, Debbie," but it touches on one of the central reasons I became a physician. I applaud the courage of the author to write about his humaneness, and I applaud *JAMA*'s courage in publishing it.

Watson Kime, M.D.

To the Editor:
I am fully aware that a physician's duty is to treat and heal, but when healing is clearly not possible, should not mercy killing be allowed? Humaneness is also a definitive part of the medical profession, and it seems that something should be done to prevent so many people from existing for sustained periods of time in a living hell. The technology we have today is wonderful, but it cannot and should not be used in every instance.

Susan D. Wilson

To the Editor:
What is more unethical, to let this young woman live in misery or to relieve her suffering?

You have to put yourself in this young woman's place and realize what she was going through before you can judge this physician for his actions.

I am a 23-year-old legal secretary and I watched my mother die of lung cancer. It was a horrible death and not one that I would like to endure myself. Cancer patients who are terminally ill endure much pain and suffering. I feel very strongly that if such a patient wants to end her life by being injected with morphine or any other drug that will end her pain, then she should have that right. No one should have the right to make someone suffer.

Diane Davis

To the Editor:
Nonmaleficence, that a physician should do no harm, was one of the first concepts introduced to us and our classmates during orientation to medical school. As physicians, we will be entrusted with the care of the human being and will continually encounter hopeless situations. Nevertheless, the role of the physician is to provide the best possible care to the patient. The taking of a life is not appropriate action for a care giver.

After the physician's emotionally detached account of the action taken to end the patient's life in "It's Over, Debbie," we realize that there are practicing physicians who either do not take the time to think of the maleficence of their actions or who are ignorant of such a notion. The resident who injected an overdose of morphine into Debbie violated the principle of "do no harm." . . .

Instead of offering a caring solution, the resident disregarded respect for human life and justified the actions on the basis of emotional frustration and limitations in technical ability. Emotion and pain endured by the patient cannot be allowed to de-emphasize the value of a human being, neither can it alter the professional responsibility of the care giver. Additionally, difficult decisions concerning treatment for the terminally ill must include the patient and personal physician, the opinion of the family, and possible review by a hospital ethics committee. . . .

In many life situations, our most important resources are not technical manuals but personal reflection and the capacity to interact with others. We cannot end a patient's life for any reason, let alone the lack of a procedural treatment. It is our hope that in times of despair we can sharpen our vision to act constructively rather than destructively. We hope to provide an environment that is appropriate for the life of the patient.

Gregory B. DiRusso
Jeffrey S. Driben
Mark R. Druffner
Roseann Lauricella
Satya Sarma

To the Editor:
Although I do not wish to condone the actions of the unnamed resident as detailed in "It's Over, Debbie," I do think it is important for the American Medical Association to consider the problems in caring for sick and dying patients, one of which is active euthanasia.

It makes no sense to hide our heads in the sand when many different forms of active euthanasia are currently being practiced in the United States. Discussing these may help bring about a social consensus that would support traditional physician reluctance to engage in active euthanasia.

Problems do exist, however, in prolonging life beyond any reasonable and comfortable limit. These problems must be thoroughly discussed by our health professional societies as well as by our citizens.

David C. Thomasma, Ph.D.


# THE IMPOSSIBLE CHOICE

## Carl M. Kjellstrand, M.D.


"No, Doc," he said, "I can't stand it anymore. No one should have pain like this and when you give me the medicines I throw up and I see things that aren't there and I'm scared to death."

He had been using the artificial kidney for five years. A proud and private man, he seemed to have no friends and did not get along well with the staff. Then he developed circulatory insufficiency, small-vessel disease, in both legs. There was nothing for the surgeons to do. When we tried analgesics we caused his nausea and changed unendurable pain to unendurable horrors of hallucinations that clouded his mind. When we treated the nausea it made the other things worse. All we could do was to amputate both legs.

He refused to have that done and decided to stop dialysis and die.

"Listen, Doc," he said. "I'm 68 years old, I live alone, and there is nothing wrong with my brain. Obviously I can't take care of myself with both legs lopped off, and being transported between a nursing home full of senile people and dialysis is more than I can take. Death is just fine with me, better than anything you can offer."

So dialysis was stopped and every day I visited him, squirming when I entered his room, where death was growing closer day by day. On the third day, just as I was leaving after a little chat, he asked me to come back.

"Doc," he said, "I still have my awful pain. You and I know that I will be gone in a week or two maybe. I'm not dumb, I understand how I'm going to go: the potassium in my blood will build up and then my heart will stop. You can't imagine what it's like, when there's no one around, to lie here and stare while life stretches the seconds and minutes to minutes and hours. I seem to have been here for years.

"See the potassium bottle over there? Please, just shoot it right into my vein. What's the difference? The potassium is going to go up and my heart is going to stop and that will be that, just similar to what will happen by itself, but it will be now and it will save me this agony of waiting and pain. I hurt when you just look at these dead legs of mine."

Already his request to stop dialysis had made us face those horrible choices of evils confronting the characters in Greek tragedies. We could stop and invite early death or we could violate his rights and go on. Both decisions were wrong: one could be seen as murder or assisted suicide, the other as assault of the strong on the weak. There was no escape; not to choose was the choice to go on, and now he made us face even more impossible dilemmas.

There were two variations of each main theme. I could comply with his request. He was right. Death would be the

same as it would be when it came by itself later. The other
extreme was to do as was done to an incompetent patient in
a New York hospital: tie him in bed and dialyze him against
his wishes and force him to take us to court to make us
stop. That seemed to be the most wrong of all the choices.
Our patient knew exactly what was going on and to violate
his or anyone's rights like that seemed a terrible violence,
although it certainly would result in the longest survival.
But he would have to bear the pain and discomfort for a
long time. Of course, as La Rochefoucauld said, "We all
have enough fortitude to take the misfortune of others."
Then there was the variation of going on. Why not simply
render him unconscious with drugs and then dialyze him?
Then we would snuff out his pain and stretch out his life.
That too has been suggested. But that was another obvious
violation of his wishes and rights, and it seemed pointless
to prolong an unconscious life. Who would benefit from
that? The fourth choice was to continue the course we were
on. We were honoring his wish to stop treatment: the ex-
pense of nameless pain was of course borne by him, but it
would be over in a week or two. I could see no other choices
than these four. In two of them you violate his rights and
extend life. In two of them you respect his rights and accept
death.

"No, John," I said. "You are asking me to do something
I believe no person should ask anyone to do: to take a human life. I cannot do that. I have three reasons: the first
one seems to me to destroy the most basic human relation.
No one should kill anyone else. Wars, electric chairs, gas,
nooses, poisons, guns—to me it's all wrong, a feeling I have
in my guts. The second reason may be a coward's. How
about if a nurse comes by and sees me? I guess I would
ultimately go free, but certainly the law would drag me over
the coals for a very long time before dropping me. So because I am scared I ask you to take the pain—not very noble! The third reason is a physician's relationship with his
patients. If physicians start to kill, then there may be no

end. Everyone would be afraid and distrustful. I can't do it.''

He started to cry, silently sobbing with tears running down his cheeks. "I'm sorry, Doc," he said. "I'm sorry I asked you."

Death was merciful to us—and maybe to him. The next day he was quite lethargic, and four days later he was found dead by a nurse. There were no signs of struggle.

# SARA

## Mark J. Pellegrino, M.D.

The morning was not going well. In the first two hours at the free-standing ambulatory clinic where I worked, 13 patients had already come in. Their ailments ranged from anterior talofibular ligament sprains to viral upper respiratory tract infections. Only a fraction of the charts had been written by the time I entered the room where the next patient awaited.

Sitting on the examination table was a young girl of about 5. She was wearing a ruffled pink dress with a large white bow tied in the front. Her hair was light brown, the color of sweet honey, with gentle curls that barely reached her shoulders. But her right hand was immersed in a bowl of Betadine, and her large brown eyes gleamed behind a thin haze of tears. When I came in, she looked a little frightened.

Standing closely beside her was a tall woman in her early 30s, her face an older, bespectacled version of the child's.

She turned to her daughter and began gesturing with her hands, synchronizing these movements with softly mouthed words: "It's all right. The doctor is here." The little girl responded with a similar fluid hand pantomime, and I realized that the mother and daughter were communicating by sign language.

"Sara is completely deaf," the mother confirmed to me. "She had meningitis when she was 6 months old."

I felt a twinge of sadness. On the outside, Sara looked like any other little girl. Yet, invisible to me, her delicate hair cells were gone, ravaged long ago. Only a nonreceptive layer of sclerosis and a silent world remained.

"We were on the way to Sara's dance class when she accidentally fell onto the gravel."

"Dance class?" I inquired, almost guiltily.

"Oh yes!" Her mother laughed at my surprise. "Sara dances to the vibrations from the music. Despite her hearing loss, she loves to do the things any 5-year-old would." She looked at Sara and signed "Dance is fun?" and a wobbly smile appeared on the child's face.

I pointed to her immersed hand, and speaking slowly, hoping she could lip-read, I told her I would fix it. She looked over to her mother, who smiled reassuringly. Sara held out her injured hand for me. There were numerous minor abrasions; nothing serious, though.

"It's OK," I said, indicating the universal "OK" with my fingers. I told her that I would clean and bandage the wounds. She nodded her head, her curls bouncing.

As I gently removed bits of embedded gravel from Sara's hand, I became sharply aware of surrounding sounds: the air conditioner whir, the telephone ring, the intercom buzz, all of which I had heard a thousand times but had always taken for granted. A door slam in the next room startled me, but Sara didn't react. She continued to gaze calmly at her hand—and then at me.

Sara watched me curiously. Although she held tightly to her mother's hand, she released her grip often to "talk."

Was her mother mad at her for falling, could she still go to dance class, and would Dad buy her ice cream tonight?

Sara's mother responded to each question with a soothing smile and tender reassurance. "No, I'm not mad," she spoke and signed. "It was not your fault. We will all get ice cream later." Their hands fluttered around each other's, almost but not quite touching.

By the time I had taped the dressings in place, Sara's eyes were no longer teary but seemed to sparkle. She tested the movements in that hand, apparently satisfied that everything still worked, then placed the tips of her right fingers against her mouth and threw them forward as if throwing me a kiss.

"That means 'Thank you,' " Sara's mother said.

I smiled at Sara and replied, "You're welcome!" Suddenly, she threw her arms around me and surprised me with a big kiss. She then bounded to the floor and skipped down the hall, swinging her purse and her mother's hand.

"Thank *you*, Sara," I thought as I watched her leave. It was going to be a good day after all, I promised, as I headed for the next room.

# ANNA, MARY, ROSE

## Michael Buenaflor, M.D.

Long before the current go-around with the federal government and at a time when young, newly trained physicians were considered poor businessmen if they did take part, I chose to be a Medicare-participating practitioner. Some of my peers had what they called "strong principles" that did not allow them to do likewise. Today I accept that I may be in the minority of physicians, but I am an old softy for my senior citizens and am proud of it.

Some doctors tried to discourage me when I chose the community in which I now practice. They felt its ethnic base, blue-collar economy, and somewhat off the beaten track location would not contribute to a successful practice. I took it as a challenge. When I opened my practice in 1979, prospective patients would walk into my office unannounced just to look around and to glimpse the new doctor. I was frequently asked whether I was a foreign doctor by elderly women wearing babushkas on their heads who, after having been in the United States for 40 years, still spoke with a heavy eastern European accent.

In the early days, with time on my hands and for convenience, I would make "house calls" at the nearby senior citizens' high rise. As I walked the hallways I would read the nameplates. For the tenants' security the doors bore no last names, only first names, which ran: Anna, Mary, Rose, Anna, Mary, Rose. There were few male residents, most having died of lung diseases associated with work in the cement mills, quarries, or mines. These surviving women had raised large families, often while working full-time in the garment mills or the local cigar factory long since closed. As a group they had invented the work ethic before there was such a term.

My calls were a grand social event. I was given a formal tour of the two-room apartment and asked to view the great-grandchildren's pictures cluttered atop the TV. My patients and I usually discussed some old piece of furniture that had graced the homes of their younger years. Such pieces would contrast sharply with the other furnishings, which resembled the complete roomsful of furniture advertised in the daily newspaper for $399. I remember a large oak dresser with fine carved legs, a marble top, and dovetailed drawers, in the corner of one apartment. The large mirror and angle of placement allowed me to observe myself and the patient from anywhere in the room as if we were watching ourselves on a large screen. That and other pieces would always remind me symbolically of Anna, Mary, and Rose—old but durable, original, valuable, full of workmanship and history, qualities most attractive to a romantic like myself.

What an experience for a young doctor! The medical portion of my visits was routine, as was my being paid. What wasn't routine was the custom some women had of kissing their doctor's hand and giving him some homemade baked goods to take along. Often someone would labor over a pot of soup to have it on hand to offer me on the first cold winter day. This was especially likely once they discovered that I made these calls on my lunch hour. I could well fantasize how wonderfully calorie-laden a barter system could be.

I don't remember if it was Anna, Mary, or Rose I admitted to the hospital one year, but on arriving home after her illness she came to my office and paid me $300 cash in small bills. I would have waited for the Medicare check but she "didn't want to accept something for nothing." Furthermore, she refused to sign a Medicare form, which would have allowed her to recover at least 80% of her money. She told me how when she came to the United States many years before, she was welcomed and given a job and had managed to have a good life. Now she felt the government needed the money more than she, and she did not intend to take any kind of charity. I was speechless.

Little has changed in my first seven years of practice. But Mary doesn't take ill at the bingo hall anymore. Rather, she suffers from one-armed-bandit bursitis of the shoulder, a consequence of her bus trips to Atlantic City with the senior citizens' club. This is progress. At Christmas she slipped an extra $20 into my pocket from her winnings. She did this with the demeanor of a loving grandmother. Sometimes, when she gets me laughing so hard, I realize that she is downright therapeutic for me, and I feel I should pay her.

Anna, Mary, and Rose have tendered as much pride to my practice as they have humility to me personally. Anna, my cleaning lady, would not accept a decent wage, because she felt that as a retired person on Social Security, she would be cheating the government by accepting money. Mary picks up the trash and pulls weeds outside my office. Rose cleans and irons my curtains. They attend church regularly and always include me in their prayers. It is often difficult to tell who is serving whom.

I know that I am the beneficiary of such kindness, not because I personally deserve it but because to Anna, Mary, and Rose I represent all the doctors they have ever known, and all the good deeds ever done for them by any doctor. I am the custodian of the trust, hard work, and the goodwill of doctors who have gone before me. Today, when a practice is transferred or sold, one physician pays another cash for "goodwill." I never had to do that, even though I share the goodwill established by my predecessors. To participate in Medicare is to accept less monetary return, but it is my way of paying my debt to those other physicians while at the same time helping my patients stretch their fixed incomes.

Clearly the ranks of senior citizens will swell in our future. This will be positive if you see senior citizens as I do for what they are, both a national and personal resource. Anna, Mary, and Rose have added a certain dignity and integrity to my practice that could be done only by those who have lived a lifetime, and whose experience and example make them a most worthwhile source of professional consciousness. The down side is that these seniors are more likely to become ill and die. I've always hated losing friends. Just the same, I'll take care of them the best I can. I'll enjoy them and reap the benefits of their soup, cookies, and loyalty, for they won't be with me forever, and I have so much left to learn from them. That may be good business or it may be bad business, but it's our business—mine and Anna, Mary, and Rose's.

# THE HYPNOTIST

## Kathleen Schneider-Braus, M.D.

They billed me as a hypnotist. Granted, psychiatrists easily slip into the realm of shamans, priests, and healers, but still it made me nervous to have the oncologists and residents promising I would deliver the magic of hypnotism. What did that mean to the young woman riddled with leukemia and needing her eighth bone marrow sampling? The last two procedures had been performed with the patient under general anesthesia because the previous five had made her famous for screaming, jumping from the bed, and other hysterics. Now the anesthesiologist was squeamish because of her compromised lung function. Too apprehensive to "snow" her with medication, and knowing it hadn't worked well in the past anyway, the team of doctors felt backed into a corner. Time to call the hypnotist.

The deck was stacked against me. The medical team received me with dubious respect and the nursing staff had a more open skepticism in their manner. The woman herself appeared pale and very near the end of her rope, but I sensed a strain of stubborn courage through the tears and despair. She told me she felt she could get through the chemotherapy, the infections, even the high risk of death—anything but the pain of the bone marrow. I admired her, mostly for her imperfect strength and her blunt humanness.

The bone marrow was to be done ASAP. If I believed the hypnosis wouldn't work after the half-hour induction, I was to call it off. The operating room was already scheduled for the next day. Beginning the induction and realizing the woman could not relax lying back because of her cough, and could not close her eyes because she was deaf and needed to read my lips, I nearly called to confirm the OR reservation. I couldn't think of a polite way to get out, so I began. I insisted she receive a tranquilizer and some morphine to increase my chances. I was, after all, trained in biological psychiatry and my confidence needed a boost.

She was a surprisingly good subject—able to warm and cool alternate hands. I motioned the team to begin. Using the 23rd Psalm as her cue, I felt the hypnosis session was more like a religious revival, holding her sweat-drenched hands, shouting to her about cool waters and green pastures, eyes locked, face to face 6 inches apart.

Then it was over. She couldn't believe it. I felt exhausted and unable to bounce back to my medical persona. The oncologist gave a sly grin and said he had a few other referrals for me. But as I walked out of the room my sense of miracle was shattered. The oncologist said, "So you call that hypnosis? Looked like relaxation to me." I admitted that I hadn't levitated anyone or pulled a rabbit from a hat, but that that was hypnosis all right. We don't really know what it is, so how could I explain it? I read his procedure note: "Bone marrow was performed with 1 mg Ativan, 4 mg morphine, and relaxation technique."

I thought a lot about what I did in that room. I doubt that it was more or different from what old-time general practitioners used to do, or midwives, or Indian medicine men. The difference lay in the skepticism of the oncologist. Hypnosis relies on the human's ability to focus and relax; it contains little iatrogenic risk and is not costly. Yet it takes a backseat to medication in the Western world's approach to patients. The reluctance to accept hypnosis may be a question of efficiency or reliability, but perhaps it's more a question of faith.

# TOMMY

## Abigail Zuger, M.D.

I'm almost sure he's dead by now; the last time I talked to
the people in New York, he had sent his family away and
was refusing to eat or open his eyes.

He wasn't particularly unique: a skinny little drug addict
with a long prison record and a fast mouth, who hadn't
managed to turn his life around in time. He was, in fact,
more or less indistinguishable from all the other patients in
our Friday morning AIDS clinic. But we all agreed that
Tommy had a certain style.

His AIDS was diagnosed about two years ago. When he
appeared in my examining room for the first time a month
later, I learned that he was married and no longer used
drugs. On his second visit he mentioned that his wife was
four months pregnant. On his third visit he confided that
she was also mentally retarded. Sandra couldn't read, write,
or travel around the city by herself, although apparently she
cooked a wicked *arroz con pollo*.

By the fourth visit I had accumulated a lot of issues to
discuss with him—but he arrived panting and febrile, and I
put him back in the hospital instead.

When he was discharged, he had no time for issues. The
relatives he and Sandra were staying with had found out
what AIDS really meant. Her father kicked them out, but
his brother took them in; then his brother kicked them out,
but his mother took them in. His mother was having second

thoughts just about the time Tommy started having problems breathing again.

He wouldn't come into the hospital until someone found a place for Sandra to stay. When the city agencies heard AIDS, they said no. She wound up on the floor next to his bed on 12 North, in terrified violation of all the rules, making her hugely pregnant self as small as possible, while Tommy's intern stood guard at the door and Tommy struggled for breath through the night.

Three weeks later, in a triumphant feat of social work, he was discharged to a rent-free city apartment. Tommy felt his luck was changing, and he began to fight. Turning on all his charm, he visited all the agencies that were doing anything at all for people with AIDS. The syndrome had just become newsworthy, and reporters flocked his way. He was featured in the *Daily News* and interviewed on the radio. He joined the AIDS support group at the hospital and suffused it with energy, visiting his new friends with food and presents when they were hospitalized, holding their hands, calling their relatives when they died.

For some reason, his own health remained good. For a while, I could see that he thought he was going to win the war against his disease. For a while, he had me believing he would too. Sandra had her baby, a fat little girl with no signs of AIDS. Tommy passed the one-year anniversary of his diagnosis. The rest of the AIDS support group slowly died off, one by one. No one formed another one.

Instead of going to the group, Tommy haunted my clinic. Every Friday morning he grinned at me from the waiting area, whether he had an appointment or not, always with a fistful of new color snapshots of the baby. I dreaded telling him I would be leaving the hospital at the end of June.

When at last I broke the news, he didn't disappoint me, moping and mourning through all my careful reassurances, losing so much weight that his cheekbones stood out like delicate wings in his drawn face. "He's just sad," I told the social worker—but, of course, I was wrong. I finally ordered a chest film, and it was clear that Tommy had lost the war.

He had visited too many friends in the hospital to have any illusions about the powers of modern medicine against his disease. He humored us by agreeing to all our diagnostic tests, but from his hospital room he made out a will and sent Sandra and the baby off to live with relatives in Puerto Rico. Until he got too weak to get out of bed, he spent his afternoons wandering through the wards—almost all the private rooms were occupied by friends of his from the clinic—chatting, explaining what a bronchoscopy was, showing his snapshots. When I came to say good-bye on my last day at work, he was asleep.

In my new hospital, AIDS is not yet a reality. It's still one of those epidemics that exist only on paper, defined by journal articles and statistics. Young people don't generally make out their wills here, or reminisce about their bronchoscopies, or go to each other's funerals. When I tell people what things are like back in New York, they smile and shake their heads.

No one wants to hear about Tommy here.

# DR. MOM

## Margaret Levy, M.D.

I am not a liberated woman. I am incarcerated in a world and life-style far more complex and complicated than my great-grandmother (raising her 11 children in an apartment in the Bronx) could have imagined. I don't care whether I am addressed as Miss, Mrs., Ms, doctor, nurse, chairman, chairperson, sir, ma'am, or hey-there. I used to become very angry when patients would call out to me, "Hey, nurse, I need a bedpan." It's far easier just to give them a bedpan.

When I was a medical student, I was naive enough to believe that I could do everything I wanted to do. I had no role model. Yes, I knew women who were physicians, even a couple of whom were surgeons. But these people were aberrations to me—unhappy, unbalanced, androgynous, and often downright hostile. Now that a decade has passed since I was graduated from medical school, I realize how impossible it is not to be one among them. It is a continuous struggle not to be. I admire those women who have totally dedicated themselves to their careers. You all know such women. Take a look at them. Now think of your male colleagues who have made major contributions in their fields, or think of those whom we label as workaholics. Notice any difference? Of course. Even the most dedicated of your male colleagues goes home to a wife and family.

Now comes the woman who thinks she can have a rewarding career in medicine and—at the same time—raise a family. Let me tell you, once and for all, that this is neither physically nor psychologically possible. The myth is that a woman engaged in a rewarding career—in any profession—can raise her children. Take my word for it, someone else is, call it Grandma, au pair girl, or day care, call it anything but Mom. Okay, so maybe she is doing it part-time: part-time Mom and part-time doc. Now her peers don't respect her (she just isn't dedicated enough) and her kids are confused and she is exhausted and angry and feels like she is copping out. Riddled with guilt lest her patients need her and she is home watching "Sesame Street" or it is Josh's first day in kindergarten and she is stuck at the hospital with a sick patient.

I have discussed these issues with dozens of women in our profession. The solution in my family has been for my husband to suspend his career to be a full-time parent so that I can be a full-time surgeon. The result of this is that I have two beautiful sons who have a unique worldview (I remember when Michael was all of 3, he asked me if men could be doctors too!). I am envious of all of the time my husband has had with the kids, and he is now struggling to get back into a career track after having been out of the "real world" for eight years. Our choice was made out of the dismay we both felt when seeing our friends' "day-care kids," who are absolutely pathetic, no matter how good the day care is. In addition, we had invested too much in my career and realistically could anticipate—at least financially—a better life-style with me as the breadwinner. Not to mention that sometimes I really do love my work.

Our solution is a rather unusual one, but I have found what I have in common with my female colleagues—being in a constant state of exhaustion and frustration. If any of you out there have fared better, I would like to hear from you.

# TWELVE BROWN EGGS

## Jack L. Mayer, M.D.

Twelve brown eggs. Every Wednesday they're on my desk like a dozen inflated pennies. Mrs. Labelle leaves them as payment on her bill in my pediatrics office on the Canadian border. She has little money but lots of chickens. In the northeast kingdom of Vermont the "economic recovery" doesn't mean much in terms of cold cash.

When I first came to this town ten years ago, filled with the romance of rural New England, I posted a sign inviting barter: "Times are tough. If you are having trouble paying your bill, I would be happy to discuss bartering goods or services." It wasn't long before Mrs. Boisonneau began crocheting a series of blankets, hats, and sweaters that far exceeded the number of beds, heads, and bodies in my family.

Anthony and Edward Delain seemed to pick up every croup, otitis, and bronchitis plaguing the county, but Mr. Delain, an independent logger with neither health insurance nor savings account, didn't like to owe anyone money.

"I know I'm behind on my bill, Doc." He shifted weight uneasily and fingered his wool cap. "Saw your sign outside. I don't got much to trade but I cut wood."

"I could use firewood. I burn about four cords a year."

"This here's my busy season, but by October I could have four cord of nice maple, birch, and elm for you." He pronounced it Vermont-style, "el-um."

I reached out my hand and we shook. "Give me a call before you come so I can tell you where to unload it. And thanks."

I could see he had something else to say but he turned to go. He took two indecisive steps and changed his mind. "I ain't got the cash to pay you and I feel real bad about it. But I cut good firewood. You won't be sorry. The boys'll want to come along. See where Dr. Jack lives. My old man, he used to tell me about tradin' with Dr. Judd but I don't know of no doctors that trade anymore."

A month after Mr. Delain and the boys delivered my firewood Brian Lussier's mother called me. It was a Monday morning in early October and the weekend on call had been beastly. The foliage had peaked a week before, and most of the leaves blew down in a blast of arctic air called the Alberta Clipper. This feels like the coldest time in Vermont. The trees and ground are as bare as an uncovered sleeper and the night frosts bring memories of last winter. People are reluctant to put on their winter coats, hanging onto fall jackets like amulets.

The first viral epidemic filled my waiting room, and I was

late because of an unscheduled C-section at the hospital 30 miles away. Mrs. Lussier didn't come very often and Brian was still behind on his shots. Jan handed me the phone as I ushered the noisy Shurtleff clan into my office.

"Hello, Mrs. Lussier? This is Dr. Mayer. What's up?"

"It's Brian. He's had a fever since last Wednesday and the Tylenol don't help. I thought he'd be better by now but he looks bad to me. Must be his ears. I was wonderin' if you could call the Rexall and give him some of that pink penicillin. It fixed him up in good shape last time."

"Mrs. Lussier, I can't prescribe an antibiotic over the phone. And it sounds like I need to see him. Is he drinking fluids?"

"Well, not real good. He just lays around and takes a sip. I think he's got a sore throat. We all been sick."

"I think you'd better bring him in this morning. Do you have transportation?"

"I could get my husband to come back from the pulp mill. But," she paused and her voice fell, "we don't have no insurance. I can't pay you."

"Doesn't matter. You pay when you can. Brian needs to be seen."

"I don't know. My husband don't like to run up bills."

"Mrs. Lussier, please. He needs to be seen."

Twenty-month-old Brian was lethargic. He sat mute and dull-eyed in his mother's lap, mouth hanging open, limbs unmoving. His temperature was 105 and his neck was stiff. When I told his mother that he might have meningitis and would need to be in the hospital, she sighed deeply and picked at her frayed coat.

"I know you're worried about Brian." I pushed the box of Kleenex to her. "He needs blood tests and a spinal tap. If he has meningitis he'll have to go to Burlington, to the medical center. He'll get the best care."

"I'll have to talk with my husband. He's waitin' in the car."

"Mrs. Lussier." It was hard to ask this question, but I had to know. "Did you wait because of the money?"

She nodded and took another tissue.

"Is that why he's behind on his shots?"

She nodded again.

Brian survived his *H influenzae* meningitis but he's in a special education class. Mrs. Lussier puts $5 toward her bill every month without fail. One day I saw her looking wistfully at my barter sign. She buys her own eggs. Her house is cold in winter.

# OUR NEW HOME

## Dena L. Lovett

We moved three months ago. My husband has a job here. He works seven days a week and he's gone all night every couple of days. I know he doesn't sleep those nights because he is so tired when he finally comes home.

I have no friends or relatives here. Many days go by when I speak to no one except my children. I've been to church, but everyone hurries home and the pastor hasn't called. I've looked hard for a job, but no one here wants or seems to need my skills.

My little girl of 3 misses her Daddy very much. She goes to preschool in the mornings. There are no children in our neighborhood. My son is just 9 months old. He doesn't miss Daddy. They don't know each other very well because Daddy is gone so much.

My husband doesn't make enough money to pay the bills. Until now we were eligible for low-interest loans. I had a job. We moved her from a small town. Our rent is more than twice as much here. I suppose we should take our daughter out of preschool; it is so expensive here. But why should she be lonely too? If I could find a job to help pay for things, maybe my husband wouldn't talk about how much better off we would be without him. He knows I could find a good job in many other places. But we love him. We can't leave.

The nights I must spend alone are the worst. There is so much crime in our neighborhood. I lie awake in fear. I keep a loaded gun in the bedroom. I fear for my children. I fear for myself.

We dreamed of being so happy in our new home. Instead, we have found fear and loneliness. We have found the nightmare of internship. Does anyone care? Will anyone help?

# MAX

## Mark S. Litwin, M.D.

I remember your hands running through my wavy hair, as we rocked away a sultry August evening. Crickets chirped through the silence of a South Carolina breeze, and Charleston seemed the safest place on earth.

Although I was the oldest of three children, at 7 I hardly understood the meaning of divorce. I was scared, but you comforted me. You held me close to your heart and protected me with the strength of your hands.

"They're made of steel," you joked, closing your fists around my tiny wrists. These were the hands of an old soul. They had supported a household of eight after your father's death during the Depression; now they were called on again to mend the hearts of three young grandchildren bewildered by the fracture of a family. Here, my education began.

"When you learn somethin', brother, you got it," you would say, tapping your index finger on a white-haired, but mostly bald, head, as we memorized together all the presidents and the capitals of all the states. You instilled deep in me a curiosity for life and a sense of independence.

I remember walking through Hampton Park to take the hot city bus downtown to your office furniture store. On top of your great steel desk was a windup bird cage that planted "Some Enchanted Evening" clearly in my memory. You taught me about music and history and art and religion. And as I grew, I learned more and more from you about compassion and people.

By the time I was 12 years old, the business had greatly expanded, yet every day after school you'd close your office door, and we'd study together as I prepared to become a Bar Mitzvah. You shared the pulpit with me when I entered manhood at 13.

In high school I took an afternoon job in the warehouse. You taught me how to haul cartons on a hand truck, how to buy merchandise, and how to sell a chair and desk to a customer who called for a file cabinet. You taught me the importance of professional integrity.

I went away to college to major in economics, intending to return and enter the family enterprise, but newfound interests led me to science. When I phoned you three years later to say I had accepted a place in medical school, I thought you would be disappointed. But you gave me your blessings and quietly rearranged your retirement from the business.

We spent the next four years learning medicine together. We explored the recesses of the human body from anatomy to neurophysiology.

During my studies of cardiovascular pathology, you suffered a heart attack. I knew enough to fear losing you, but not enough to anticipate your recovery. As you lay sedated in the intensive care unit, the cardiac monitor chirping through your silence, I took your hand in mine. Although your body lay flaccid, the strength in your fingers gave me fortitude to weather the crisis.

Twenty years after we began, you continue to teach me. As I endure the rigors of my surgical residency, you still send me newspaper clippings, speech reprints, and magazine subscriptions, constantly exposing me to new disciplines inside and outside the scope of medicine. I have studied under many renowned professors during these last several years. You never graduated college, but you are my greatest teacher.

Last week, I visited a patient's room to remove several silk sutures before leaving the hospital after 48 hours on duty. I struggled to keep my eyes open. When I finished, I noticed tears in the gentleman's eyes. The reality of his cancer had struck him. He was your age, but his hands were wizened and drained of their vitality. I sat at his bedside and took his hand. As I spoke to him, I looked down and saw in my hands the strength of yours. I held him tightly and encouraged him to express his sadness until he felt better.

When I arrived home I cried too. I thought of you and the gift you have given me. Others taught me to auscultate, but you taught me to listen. Others taught me to close incisions, but you taught me to heal patients. Others are teaching me to operate with my hands, but you gave them their strength.

My hair now adorns mostly the back of my head, and I feel more like you each day. From heart to hands and hands to heart, you have taught me to be a physician. Thank you.

# DADDY'S LITTLE GIRL

## Ida M. Onorato, M.D.

"He's not doing too well today," my mother said. "I'm not sure he'll know you. But try to talk to him anyway."

It was five years ago that I spoke to my father on the phone and knew something was wrong. As always, he was very interested in my work. I was telling him about my new research project and he asked, "DTP—is that for whooping cough?" A general practitioner for 40 years, he had probably given thousands of DTP shots to "his babies" (as he used to call them). I talked to my mother. "Has Daddy had a checkup lately? Have you noticed anything wrong? Do you think he is getting a little forgetful?" His son, the psychologist, thought he was depressed. "After all, he's not used to being retired. He misses his patients; he doesn't have enough to do. Maybe an antidepressant would help." But his daughter, the internist, knew better. After all, I have always been my father's child.

The first Halloween costume I remember was a nurse's uniform. Growing up in the 1950s, I wanted to be a nurse. Daddy and I made house calls together, driving into the country in the late afternoon dusk after school, while my younger brother, "the baby," and my mother stayed home and made dinner. Almost every house we visited had milk and cookies for me and often cake, eggs, or chickens for my daddy. I could answer the phone in Daddy's office downstairs in our big house and tell patients that "the doctor is on a maternity'' years before I understood what the words meant. Sunday afternoons after church Daddy and I went to the hospital to make rounds on his patients. I played in the nurses' station and sometimes, awed by the shiny equipment and hushed atmosphere, I was called into a hospital room to cheer up patients who had known me since I was born. At my medical school graduation 20 years later, some still remembered me making the rounds of my father's waiting room, asking them to stick out their tongues, prescribing penicillin shots, and dispensing Band-Aids from my play doctor's bag.

And so, it was inevitable that I would become a physician and inevitable that I would first diagnose my father's illness. During the x-rays and blood tests and CT scans, the rest of the family was optimistic. ''He's just getting older, everyone becomes a little forgetful when he gets older.'' My father was confused. ''Do you think there's something wrong with me? I feel OK. I'm just a little tired, that's all.'' My father's internist and neurologist, old friends of the family, hedged their bets. ''It's really a diagnosis of exclusion. We'll just have to see how he does over the next few years.'' But I knew. With the objectivity of a scientist and the intuition of a clinician, I knew. And I wished I did not know.

My father and I had talked only about the excitement of practicing medicine, the satisfaction of helping people, and the intellectual stimulation of solving problems. We had never talked about the loss of innocence that changed my perceptions of the world forever. We had never talked about how certain knowledge would set me apart from my family and others I loved, and would deprive me of the denial that has been everyone else's defense against our family's tragedy. Now we will never talk of these things. But I think my father would say that for him the joys of practicing medicine far outweighed the disadvantages. For myself, I am not so certain. During these last years, as the physician in the family I have had the responsibility of answering my mother's questions with both shaded truths and reassuring lies, and of encouraging my father when I knew there was no hope.

"Someone wants to talk to you." I heard my mother's voice in the distance as she wheeled my father to the telephone.

"Who's that? Who's there?" my father asked in a querulous voice.

"It's me, Daddy," I said. "It's your little girl."


# A DEATH IN THE FAMILY

## Lawrence R. Ricci, M.D.


On August 24, 1982, at 3:13 AM in a large metropolitan teaching hospital, my father, at the age of 72, died of complications from diffuse histiocytic lymphoma. During his brief hospitalization, we, his family, experienced his leaving the modern American way: an odd mixture of cold lighting, bright machinery, and rare, unexpected warmth.

My first glimpse of my father in the hospital startled and humbled me. One month before, he had been a fully functional, retired machinist. Since then, cancer, malnutrition, and dehydration had transformed him into an invalid. A screen exists between the way we see ourselves and our loved ones and how modern medicine sees us. I recall my confused and saddened brother describing how a nurse had asked him if our father could *walk* when he had been home.

For the most part, his physicians were competent. To me they were deferential; to my family, condescending. Teaching hospital medicine—the trickle of diagnosis, the flood of therapy, agonizing waits for prognosis, headlong therapeutic adventures, students, residents, attendings, surgeons, internists, hematologists, oncologists, nephrologists—even I couldn't keep it all straight.

Some memories pain me more than others: the angry, impatient surgical resident who wouldn't understand my frightened mother's indecision about a minor surgical procedure; the enthusiastic medical student who asked excitedly if I had palpated my father's abdominal mass; the uncertain medical resident who asked my opinion of Dad's BUN and blood sugar, who asked if I concurred with the insulin drip calculations. How could I answer these questions? I'm not this patient's doctor, I'm his son.

One memory was not as painful. A resident from India came in on his night off to see my father because, he said, he was reminded of his own father. He reviewed the medical record, spoke with us, listened to our concerns, and offered encouragement. US residents, perhaps more technically advanced but seemingly colder, wouldn't do that. US medical students might. But somewhere in the transition from fatigue and degradation to skill and confidence, from student to physician, we defer compassion, put it aside, often forever.

A corps of nurses, ranging from the least skilled aide to the most skilled postgraduate diplomate, buttress modern medical science. I recall only fleeting views of many strangers: one nurse forced me to leave my father's bedside after I had traveled 500 miles to see him so she could administer an enema on schedule; another nurse, when I requested pain medication for my dad, impatiently replied that it wasn't time yet, adding as she quickly turned to chart her notes, "Anyway, the pain med will drop his blood pressure again." Exhausted and afraid, I stood silently at her desk. Drop his blood pressure? Again? I don't understand. Is my father dying? Will you please stop writing and talk to me, stop talking and listen to me? If I, a physician, didn't understand, how much less did my family understand? What about families with no knowledgeable relative to intercede and interpret?

The final day. Code 99. Did the nurse pressing her weight

into his chest know him? Did the resident touching 400 joules to his heart know him? Did he remind them of their own? Did they touch his body with respect? Nearing the end . . . his pupils fixed and dilated . . . his skin cool and mottled . . . his heart beating but his spirit dead. I clutched at a crumpled ECG strip, the rising and falling electrical imprint, found lying in his room, now in my wallet pressed behind his 1942 photo by a tent in North Africa.

The final memory, the best one, was of a neurologist, holding my mother's hand, gazing into her eyes, whispering of primal cells, preconsciousness, and the end of purposeful life. She could not have understood much of what he said, yet she knew. She knew unmistakably the language of his heart and the syntax of his tears. I remain grateful to that healer.

As my father lay brain dead, only then did the medical forces of comfort and caring mobilize themselves. Nurses and doctors approached to console us. Their aid by then was unnecessary. We knew what had happened. We knew what was required of us. We had mobilized our own resources. Six hours later, my father died.

I believe I am a competent, caring physician, often afraid, sometimes callous, rarely petulant and childish. I hope I can hold on to the memory of my father's death, not only for myself, not only for my father, but for my craft, for my patients.

# NEXT PATIENT

## W. Blake Rodgers

It was hot, 100° at least outside, and in the 6-by-6-ft sheet cubicle I called an office, it was 106°. I know because that's what my thermometer said every time I picked it up. 106° and no windows. It was hot. I stepped into the hallway to pick up the next patient's chart. Reaching for it, I noticed the concentric stains that started under my arms had disappeared behind my tie. It was hot—the kind of heat we'd get in lower Alabama, the kind of heat that made kids fidgety and adults grumpy, the kind of heat you spent half your patient time complaining about. It was hot.

The "doctor" is getting grumpy, too. Next patient. "Doctor," because I was in name only. Actually I was a first-year medical student working in Alabama with a student group that provided free medical screening to anyone who would put up with the heat, the humidity, and the wait. A lot of people did. The "doctor" is getting grumpy, too. It's 3:30 and he hasn't had lunch. He's seen enough patients in that little cubicle today to never again want to be in a 6-by-6-ft space with another sweating body. I looked at the next chart. Age: 66. Height: 70″. Weight: 255. Great, another big, sweaty body. The doctor is getting grumpy, too.

It's tough in small towns in lower Alabama. It gets hot in April; it stays hot all summer and most of the fall; there never seems to be a break: no air-conditioning, no fans, and few, if any, windows. It's tough in small towns in lower

Alabama. Especially if you're black. Especially if you can
remember other times. And even if you can't. I was born
and grew up in the South and I figured I'd seen racism in
just about every shape and size. Then I went to school up
North and learned there were a couple of other shapes and
sizes; but hatred is still hatred, blindness, still blindness.
Or so I thought. I'd never seen anything like the horrid,
vicious face that racism wore in that little town. I'd never
been to any place where 90% of the people lived in almost
complete subservience to the other 10%. I'd never had a
103-year-old woman refuse to answer me in any way but
"yessuh" or "nossuh." I'd never seen a grown man treat
children like animals. It's tough in small towns in lower
Alabama.

I reacted badly. I'm not a diplomatic person; I'd rather
shout than discuss, fight than reason. About six hours after
we'd arrived and set up our tent clinic in the grammar
school, I was ready to fold it all up and go home. I saw the
conditions in the town, heard the rules we were told we had
to follow, and watched the light dim in some of my friends'
eyes. I reacted badly. I wanted to tell the powers-that-were
where to get off. I wanted to scream. I was angry and
ashamed: angry at what I saw and ashamed for my race and
of my race. In my haste to be zealot—a martyr—I lost all
sense of timing. We couldn't stay there; we had to get out.
I reacted badly.

Next patient. It had been four days and I was still steam-
ing. Sure, the kids in town had started to play with us. Sure,
I'd seen the fear in a child's eyes melt into a smile by giving
him a penlight. Sure, I'd given away a case of penlights.
It's not such a bad trade—a case of penlights for a case of
smiles. Next patient. I was hot and tired and still self-
righteously determined that we had to be more vocal, that,
damn the consequences, we had to establish once and for
all where we stood, that we had to be sure that they knew
we weren't just like people from around there. Next patient.

"Mr. Johnson." Mr. Ezekiel Johnson. "Yessuh." "Hi,
my name's Blake Rodgers and I'm a medical student. Could

you please step back this way? Been hot enough for you?''
''Yessuh.'' Mr. Johnson. He looked heavier than 255, older
than 66. He was only 3 inches shorter than I, but with my
youth and his weight, I towered over him. Light-gray hair
topped dusty brown skin that stood dark against a tan shirt,
more sweat-stained than mine. A big, hard, farm-laborer's
hand enveloped the puny response it was offered. One of
his front teeth was gone. Mr. Johnson.

His physical was pretty typical. Family medical history?
''Ain't nobody ever been sick much.'' Personal health? ''I
ain't never had no problems what I couldn't take care of.''
How do you feel today? ''Well, suh, I feel a little run down,
kinda tired like, but I 'magine it's the heat.'' He smoked,
drank ''a little bit now and again,'' could stand to lose 50
to 60 pounds. Blood pressure, 165/90; temperature 99°
(second attempt; the first time the thermometer read 106°);
lungs, ''a little tight'' (or at least that's what I said; I always
heard lung ''tightness'' when I wanted someone to stop
smoking). Sadly, his physical was pretty typical.

Very typical really. He and I started by measuring each
other, trying to find out if the other could be trusted. He
started out by not looking at me, I by requesting that he not
call me ''sir.'' We talked about his children and he looked
at my face. We talked about how his wife of 45 years had
died of a heart attack two years previously and he looked at
the floor, still grieving. I grieved. We talked. We listened.
I complained about his blood pressure and his smoking. He
promised to have the blood pressure checked at the nearest
clinic. He complained that a man his age couldn't quit
smoking. We talked. We listened. We disagreed.

He was about to leave, putting back on his shirt. I was
sitting at the table's edge making notes on his chart. He had
been a patient like any other, or unlike any other, I had
seen. I had enjoyed talking with him.

Maybe the heat had softened us—being as we were both
stuck in it and suffering through it—and maybe we had a
little bit in common, since the only air-conditioned corner
of that inferno was the office of the principal, an old, evil

mound of white man no more likely to invite Mr. Johnson
for a cold soda than he was likely to ask that "damn troub-
lemakin' Yankee med student" over to call on his daughter.

We were leaving the still sweltering cubicle. He turned.

"I sho' am glad you white folks is talkin' to us. None of
the ones around heh will. It gets rough around heh. I'member 20 years ago, they cut off a man's ear and made him
chew on it up there in the center of town. Things ain't
changed much. I sho' am glad you white folks is talkin' to
us."

He turned to leave. I choked, mumbled something about
change coming, slowly but surely. He grabbed my hand. He
looked me full in the eyes, squeezed my hand, and left.

I went looking for more penlights.


# THE SAINT

## C. L. Frost, M.D.


After four months, Christine had become a fixture in our
hospital—a frail, stooped figure who appeared punctually,
at 9 o'clock each morning, on the neurological ward. She
was only 35, but misfortune had already given her a world-
weary, haggard look. The faded jeans sagging around her
wasted thighs, the scuffed gray sneakers covering her drag-
ging feet, and her deep-set eyes put one in mind of an or-
phan. Beneath her limp black hair, her features at times
assumed an imperturbably ascetic appearance and, at other
times, the careworn look of someone who longed only for
reprieve.

"And how is Father today?" she'd ask, in a thin but hopeful voice.

Always, the answer was the same—silence. Father hadn't changed, could never change. Everyone knew that he could never get better.

"I've brought some food for him," she'd say, glancing toward the door of room 409. "A thermos of hot chicken broth, some homemade chocolate pudding, hand-squeezed orange juice. Father's always liked juice." Her gnarled, undersized hands, clutching a large straw basket packed with jars of pureed fruits and vegetables, would tremble slightly.

Always, the door to room 409 was shut. Even the most dedicated nurses scurried in and out as quickly as possible. The intern, who had read *House of God*, muttered that the old man was "only a gomer"—why couldn't he be transferred back to the nursing home? The attending physician avoided the room, for Christine's father was a lost cause, not someone whom he could save with his celebrated therapeutic skills. Each morning, he would merely ask if the old man's condition had improved and nod, with resigned indifference, when the intern invariably said "No."

Each morning, Christine found her father lying in bed, his head propped up by three pillows to prevent aspiration. His edentulous mouth gaped so that saliva drooled continuously down his fissured lower lip, flakes of dried milk spotted his jaw and collar, and splotches of orange juice stained his shirt. Whenever anyone entered the room, he merely blinked instinctively—recognizing no one, not even his daughter.

Christine would pull a sterling spoon from her basket, wipe it with her handkerchief, then thrust it—scooped high with chocolate pudding—into her father's open mouth.

"Here, Papa," she'd urge. "I know you can swallow. You don't need a feeding tube like they say! You can do it—just try hard. Give it all you've got!"

With a moist sponge, she'd wipe the dried milk from his chin. Often, she'd remove his old, food-splattered shirt, then reclothe him in a newly laundered, pressed one brought from home. She'd draw an ivory comb from her purse and part his hair neatly on one side. She'd shave his cheeks and chin until they were as smooth as a boy's. Sometimes, she'd even pull an old storybook from her basket—one she'd found in the attic that was filled with the illustrated fairy tales she'd enjoyed as a youngster.

"Listen, Papa," she'd coo imploringly, "I'm going to read to you. Listen, maybe if you hear these words over and over, then you'll begin to remember . . . some faint glimmer will come back!" But Father never spoke, never nodded to indicate that he understood. He just gaped.

Physicians and nurses, entering room 409 shortly after Christine's departure, would find the old man sleeping peacefully, his thin hair parted meticulously to one side and his pressed shirt looking as neat as a corporate executive's. Any moment, one imagined, he might awaken, flick on the TV, and engage a passerby in a political debate. Christine the wonderworker, it always seemed, had miraculously rejuvenated his mind and body.

Everyone marveled at this daughter who, with tireless devotion, brought homemade puddings and freshly laundered shirts and who stayed, from morning to night, talking or reading to an old man with terminal Alzheimer's disease.

"She must be a saint," said one nurse.

Everyone nodded. There was no other explanation.

A month later, two women were seen walking slowly away from room 409. One, a plump lady whose face was red and bloated, leaned against her companion and nervously dabbed her eyes. The other, a frail woman with pinched lips and drawn cheeks, embraced the stout lady with one arm, to support and console her. At the end of the corridor, the thin woman sighed deeply and her quivering lips turned up involuntarily at the corners; then a long, shrill laugh—like the roar of a volcano releasing the tension that had built up for decades within the earth's bowels—exploded down the hall.

"Who's the heavy woman, the one who's sobbing?" asked one nurse. "I don't recall seeing her here before."

"That's Christine's sister—Nancy. Their father just died," the ward doctor answered solemnly.

"Died!" the nurse exclaimed. "And Christine laughs? She can't have loved her father much if she laughs at his deathbed!"

"On the contrary," the doctor replied, "she loved him too much. For three years she cared for him like a mother—spoon-feeding him, talking to him when no one else would. Now, perhaps, she needs to laugh."

The nurse shrugged and, glancing at the two women, looked very perplexed.

# A DIP IN THE POOL

## Robert W. Marion, M.D.

Arriving at the hospital, I viewed the madhouse that was the pediatric ER with ambivalence: on the one hand, I was happy I'd be in clinic that morning; on the other, I knew that starting at 1 PM, I'd be in charge of this insanity and that my shift wouldn't end until 4 AM, when things had calmed down enough for the night float to have a better than even chance of surviving until the next morning. Spotting Phyllis, that very night float, I approached and asked, "How're you doing?"

Looking frazzled, she stared at me. "I hate this place!" she said, as she sat down. "This is the first time I've sat down since 2 AM. The paramedics brought in a couple of sisters who got burned. The 2-year-old was DOA and the 4-year-old was in shock. We worked on her for an hour but she was too far gone. I declared her at 3:30. By then, there were 20 charts in the box. I've been trying to catch up ever since.''

"How'd they get burned?" I asked.

"Bed caught fire. Their heat had been turned off and the mother had this old space heater. They were all in one bed. The mother died in the adult ER."

This story was all too familiar—kids suffering because of what the Bronx had done to them. Able to offer her nothing else, I handed Phyllis a cup of coffee and headed toward the clinic. I was the pool resident that morning. It was my job to see any child who hadn't previously been followed in our clinic. There were only three pool patients scheduled, a family of two girls, 8 and 11 years old, and their 14-year-old brother. I felt relieved; I knew I'd have time to rest before starting my marathon session in the ER.

The children were accompanied by their mother, Mrs. Ayala, a short, heavy-set, sad-eyed woman. She told me her kids had not been to a doctor in two years.

"We used to go to a private man on Fordham Road," she said, "but I have no money for that anymore. I brought them today because they need a checkup."

I nodded and began. I had learned to start with the youngest. Her name was Rosa, and she was the beauty of the family, with big brown eyes and a smile warm enough to melt snow. I took a history, did a full exam, and found nothing wrong. I planted a tine test, made a note to get a CBC and urinalysis, and looked at my watch. It was 9:40. Right on time.

Brenda, the 11-year-old, was next. Much plainer than Rosa, Brenda looked somewhat overweight and didn't smile at all. I got her up on the table and began to take the history.

"Has Brenda been in good health?"

"She's had too many bellyaches lately," the mother replied very quietly.

"Recurrent abdominal pain," I thought. She was just the right type for it: overweight, unhappy, pubescent—features I'd seen over and over again in girls who complained of bellyaches. As I glumly thought through the workup I'd have to do and the speech I'd have to deliver, I began to examine Brenda.

But when she removed her clothes I realized Brenda's problem wasn't psychosomatic. She wasn't just plump: her abdomen was protuberant, but her extremities were thin. I felt a sinking feeling as, with her lying flat, I palpated the top of her uterus, 5 cm above her umbilicus.

I quietly groaned. The sledding gets pretty rough when you're dealing with an 11-year-old who's 25 weeks pregnant. I started to fill out her chart. After Brenda was fully clothed, I said, "Mrs. Ayala, would you mind if we sent the children out for a while? We need to talk." She didn't object and the children were dismissed.

"Uh . . . has Brenda begun to get her period yet?" I asked.

"She got her first one six months ago," she answered. "None since."

"Has she . . . does she have a boyfriend?"

"No," Mrs. Ayala said quietly. And then there was silence.

I took a deep breath. "Mrs. Ayala, Brenda's about six months pregnant."

The woman didn't seem to be surprised. "I know she is pregnant," she softly said. "I've seen her clothes get tight. I know when a woman is with child."

"Why did you wait so long to come here?"

She shrugged, and tears began to fill her eyes. "All my life I've worked," she said. "I've tried to make a good life for my children, to do good for them. I see what's happening in the streets, all the drugs and the stealing. I've told my children to stay away from it but what can I do, I'm away at work all day. My girls, they're good, they listen, but my son, he thinks he doesn't need to listen to his mother, he gets mixed up with a bad crowd, and gets into trouble. So I hit him and I threaten him, I tell him I'll kill him if he gets into trouble again. And finally he listened to me, he started coming home right after school. And then, this . . .'"

Unable to continue, her eyes now filled with tears, she finished by gesturing toward the ceiling.

I hesitated, trying to understand. "You mean your son . . . ?" I asked, but she could say no words. She only cried. "It may be too late to legally do an abortion," I continued after about a minute, "but under the circumstances . . ."

"She cannot have an abortion," the mother interrupted. "It is a sin—murder. She will have the baby and I will bring it up as my own child."

"But her brother. . . . There's a good chance the baby will be abnormal."

"What my son did was a sin but it is done. This sin I can do something about."

"Mrs. Ayala, maybe if you speak to your priest."

"Doctor, we have to do what we have to do."

We spoke for over two hours. I told her of the danger to Brenda, of the harmful effect this could have on Rosa. We discussed the legal implications: her son had sexually abused Brenda, a criminal offense, and it was my duty to report the incident to the Bureau of Child Welfare. Mrs. Ayala pleaded with me not to turn the boy in, to leave the disciplinary action to her. Realizing that he needed intensive, professional help, I told her I'd hold off if she'd talk with the clinic's psychiatrist that morning, and make it her business to bring the boy for however many visits the psychiatrist felt he needed. She agreed and we both decided that it was time to end and that the boy would return another day for his physical exam. I gave Mrs. Ayala my home phone number in case she needed to talk, knowing she'd never use it. I handed her a note to take to the appointment desk at the prenatal clinic, and finally, I walked the family over to the psychiatrist's office. Saying good-bye, I doubted if I'd ever see any of them again.

After they were gone, I sat back in my desk chair reflecting on the events of the morning. The Ayalas and the girls who had died in the ER weren't unusual. Our patients lived in buildings with no heat, hot water, or electricity; they ate the lead paint chips that fell from the walls; their only pets were the rats who ran freely through their bedrooms; they watched junkies shoot up and die before their eyes, on the stoops and in the alleyways; they sweltered in summer and froze in winter. And it was our job, the pediatric staff, to keep them healthy in spite of it all, an exhausting and frustrating task.

I sat on that chair thinking about all this for an hour after they had gone. Then I went up to the ER, and started attacking the pile of charts.

# THE BARTERED BRIDE

## John J. Dempsey, M.D.

When Daniel asked me to see his sick mother I wanted to refuse. I didn't suspect subterfuge. There were many reasons for my not wanting to go. His village was 25 miles south of our research station. The heat was equatorial. The road was only a track that had never been worth much, having become worse since civil disobedience had increased. Men and equipment previously used to keep the road passable were now needed for military purposes.

Moreover, there was some concern for both protocol and safety. We were not supposed to travel without official approval, yet having escort was no guarantee against injury. An American under escort in the same area had lost an arm in an ambush a few months earlier.

Nevertheless, I went. A week earlier I had refused to make a shorter journey to see a sick daughter of one of our workers. The following day her father asked me if he could have a few hours off to bury his child. Guilt is a great prod.

The trip progressed without incident through seared, flat savanna where the heat made everything shimmer. The drought-ridden landscape seemed barren of everything but people. We were soon beyond the last sagging electric wire, beyond the last building made of anything but mud and straw, beyond where we could expect to see government personnel.

The village was clean. There were a few starving dogs but the children still had some fat on them. The long-horned cows were painfully thin, but must have remained objects of pride and beauty to the cattle-herding villagers. The *tukl* I was taken to was spotless. It boasted a screen over the low doorway through which we stooped to enter.

An old woman sat on the floor in the center of the hut. I couldn't find anything wrong with her. Daniel, acting as interpreter, was becoming impatient. We stepped outside.

Daniel seemed perfectly happy with my negative findings. What he wanted now was for me to go with him to see his cow. Apparently the cow was seriously ill and badly needed professional attention. It occurred to me that the sick cow was probably the reason for my visit.

I told Daniel that my seeing the cow would serve no purpose. I didn't even know how to go about examining a cow. I knew nothing about the diseases of the local cattle except what I had learned from the government veterinarian, that tuberculosis and brucellosis were common. He was constantly frustrated in his attempts to procure milk samples to help in epidemiologic studies and therapy. He was denied access to the herds because, as an Arab official of the government, he was not trusted.

The tribesmen were convinced that the Arabs, former slavers, were now determined to suppress and eliminate the southern tribes. To them an Arab was likely to be engaged in a clever scheme to make all those cows go dry by offering the milk to menstruating women. This would be catastrophic since the tribes' existence centered on their cattle.

Daniel and I started our journey back to town. Perhaps I seemed a bit chagrined, for he explained why the loss of this particular cow would mean so much to him.

The cow was with calf. This increased her value but was not Daniel's main concern. The real problem was that the cow was not his but belonged to his father-in-law.

A year before, Daniel had purchased his bride at a price of four cows. He had had only three animals at the time, but his prospective father-in-law was willing to give his daughter in marriage with the understanding that the remainder of the bride price would be forthcoming. Daniel subsequently purchased a cow who became with calf. His father-in-law was willing to wait until the calf was born before claiming the cow.

Things were working out nicely. The new wife fit in well in Daniel's village. She soon became pregnant and had recently been delivered of a healthy child. It looked as if Daniel would end up with wife, child, and calf. All of this came crumbling down with the illness of the cow.

It would have been foolish to try to console Daniel, who certainly knew far better than I the importance of the bride price. In such a harsh land the tribes would long ago have ceased to exist were brides not worth a great deal.

Boys become useful at a very early age since they can hunt, fish, and tend cattle long before they reach puberty. Girls are of little value until they are old enough to become mothers. Consequently, in a land of always precarious food supply, little girls would not get enough nourishment to survive in sufficient numbers to maintain tribal strength unless they were given added value. That value is the bride price.

That Daniel could buy a bride with only four cows was an indication of the relative poverty of his tribe at the time. Among wealthier groups a bride could cost as much as 20 head of cattle. A high bride price was essential. If the price were to go below the cost of keeping a daughter until she was eligible for marriage, then female infant mortality would soar and the tribe would dwindle. That this had not happened over hundreds of years in one of the most difficult terrains on the face of the earth said a great deal about the merits of the system. So deeply ingrained was the concept of the bride price that although there were a good number of native priests (including the Bishop), there were few native nuns since the church did not feel it proper to pay a bride price.

The cow died. My not seeing it had nothing to do with that outcome so my conscience wasn't troubled. I did feel sorry for Daniel. I suspected that his father-in-law felt he had already bent tribal custom as far as he could. Even if he were so inclined he would probably not be in a position to be lenient any longer.

A few days later I heard someone calling from outside our quarters. Daniel's wife had come to say good-bye. She was carrying their child. She had come the 25 miles from Daniel's village, walking barefoot in a climate so hot that I routinely found my clinical thermometers at 107 degrees, the height of the mercury column.

She didn't tarry. It was another 40 miles to her father's village. She had a long way to go.


# SELF-DEFENSE

## Sara Jo Friedman

Coffee cup in hand, 3 × 5 cards spread across the desk before me, I sit awaiting my 2 AM second wind. I am at the stage in my career in which the mystery of the next admission and the romance of medicine have not yet been overtaken by the weariness so many others describe: I like these hours best. Now is when I get the feel of this big-city hospital and the strength of the house staff who "man" it. How I look up to them, hard and cold as they are. They get the job done. They have no choice.

The intern I am following—as a third-year medicine clerk—strides in. He's pepped up on the responsibility and can't sit still: there's one more lab report to be checked, two more blood samples to be drawn. He's like a shark, constantly moving even when asleep. I force him to sit, to take his stethoscope from around his neck, and to rest. He looks so uncomfortable doing nothing.

"Hellooo-oo . . ." An echoing, plaintive call startles us. Without even looking we both know who's yelling. The intern doesn't move or comment. How he can just sit there—unmoved by the desperate voice—eludes me. For the fifth time I want to know that this time the wolf is not at this man's door. For the fifth time tonight his condition is unchanged.

The previous September he had noticed some bumps near his eyes. Now, in February, he has large, fragile vascular lesions that cover his body. He was admitted for anemia from all the blood he lost through them. He's frightening to look at; he no longer appears human. His eyes are forced shut by the lesions. He's been put in a room by himself, the first time I've seen a private room at this hospital of open wards, because the blood that is leaking from every inch of his body is a hazard. He has AIDS.

The first week I cared for him I tried to change his world. I brought him ice, and cookies I had baked at home. I encouraged him to drink his Ensure. My intern kept his distance while I tried not to keep mine. Every instinct I had drove me away from this horrifying man, but I fought myself, thinking that if I am not here for this man who needs my humanity, who am I here for?

The second week I drifted further away from him, filling my time with other patients, seeing him only when I had to. Now that he is isolated, no one goes near him. The ice bucket for the floor is outside his door, yet no one will bring him ice. The x-ray technician finds excuses for his portable films to be taken on someone else's shift. He has become a difficult patient. He screams all day and all night, always the same cry, unchanged and unceasing: "Hellooo-oo, is anyone there?" He wants ice. He wants to be told there is hope for him. He wants understanding and compassion.

Medically we have nothing to offer him. His wife cannot face taking him home, and so he remains here under our "protective custody." His daughter is the only visitor I see. She dons gloves and a gown to enter his room, but cannot bring herself to touch him. How this dread disease violated this family seems unimportant, yet this 14-year-old must wonder. I can only hope her family will survive this, even if her father won't.

And now, at 2 AM, I hear him calling out "Hellooo-oo!" and I know that his voice will haunt me long after he is gone. And I wonder if the others have escaped this spell.

The most difficult thing for me to learn is to be hardened but sympathetic, detached yet warm. How I admire the interns. How I fear losing my compassion while becoming one of them.

# CUSTODIAN

## Victor T. Wilson, M.D.

This patient, this beautiful 4-year-old boy, was brought in by helicopter from the scene of a head-on auto collision. The nurse recounts the familiar story: an unrestrained back-seat passenger, found under the front dash in the crushed plastic and steel mess. He was extracted with pneumatic jaws and immobilized on a board. Ringer's lactate brought the blood pressure up. Oxygen through an endotracheal tube pinkened his lips. He did not move then and does not now. His pupils do not shrink from light. His skull is in pieces and his brain on CT scan is distorted, cut by white jags of hemorrhage. The flurry of deep-line placements, roentgenograms, burr holes, and blood tests have settled into routine intensive care. Pressor drips infuse. His vital signs are stable now.

Bandaged and crying, his parents are led to him. Their shock, guilt, and grief are the same as they are every time, with every child like him, but still I must turn away from it. I think of my own sweet son and feel dread.

The neurological examination remained barren throughout the night: no reflexes, no tone, and no brain-stem signs. I remove his ventilator briefly and wait for him to breathe. He does not. This morning the unassailable judgment of a cerebral perfusion scan is accomplished. The boy is dead.

This is where my job usually ends. Tubing would be disconnected, machines turned off. The coroner would come. But now we ask gently and urgently of his parents that they give a great gift. Would they donate his organs? At first they are repulsed. Then their anger melts and they see in it a hope and a comfort. They whisper, and embrace, and agree.

I check on the other patients in the unit. The teenager with asthma is better. I kid him about his tattoo and he grins. The baby recovering from repair of a heart defect is not ventilating well. After some adjustments she breathes easier and grabs my finger.

A curious feeling takes me: as physician to these other children, I continue to work, hoping they will get better, that we will best the disease. But for the dead boy there is no hope and no struggle. For him I am now merely custodian of organs.

The transplant surgeons arrive. Is the heart still good? A last diagnostic flourish of echocardiogram, Swan-Ganz catheter, and isoenzymmes suggests it is. The ward clerk wonders how to bill the child's supplies, now that he is no longer a patient. His blood pressure falls slowly. A little fluid, a little more pressor drip, and he is nudged back to a tenuous homeostasis. I stand at the bedside and touch his warm toes. "He is gone, isn't he?" his mother asks. I tell her yes.

Potential recipients rush to the hospital. Heart, kidneys, eyes, and pancreas will be harvested. His parents have said their good-byes and have gone. I sit in his room and watch him, looking for the difference, but he still looks like a live little boy. In midafternoon he is wheeled past me to the operating room, the beautiful dead boy I cared for today. His vital signs are stable.

# MY FRIEND

## Thomas J. Poulton, M.D.

Brett is intensely curious about the rapidly enlarging world about him. His probing curiosity about life stimulates the adults around him to inquire more actively about their own lives. He is like most other 3-year-olds, I think: full of delightful mischief, granting smiles without hesitation and rapidly retreating to tears at those times when life is just too much bigger than he is. And, like many children, he cannot conceal a certain charming, if smug, satisfaction as he masters each new developmental task. Those tasks often come hard for Brett.

Brett has many other friends. Some, such as I, are new friends. Others, such as Grandma, Grandpa, and Daddy, go way back to before the accident that he now pretends not to remember. The accident? Brett's mother and baby brother, Matthew, were killed by a drunk driver in a violent accident on a softly beautiful starlit evening last summer. I did not know the driver, but I know he had spent the day enjoying a party with friends and relatives. It was a day of happiness and sharing, of warmth and camaraderie. It was also a day of drinking.

I grew up in a home in which the consumption of alcohol was uncommon, but not condemned. Nevertheless, the importance of responsibility and the possible adverse consequences of drinking and driving were emphasized. I can still easily recite a litany of facts about alcohol consumption and driving: a quarter of a million Americans have died in alcohol-related accidents in the last decade; one American life is lost every 20 minutes in an alcohol-related accident; half of all Americans will be involved in an alcohol-related accident during their lifetimes; alcohol-related crashes are the leading cause of death among Americans between the ages of 16 and 24 years; 2000 persons are injured each day in alcohol-related accidents; 2 million drunk-driving collisions occur each year; 80% of Americans drive after drinking; drunk drivers cost US taxpayers in excess of $20 billion annually; only about one in 1000 drunk drivers on the road is arrested. I knew all this, but I really did not know anything about the human cost of drunk driving until I met my new friend Brett.

At least one person told the drunk driver he ought not drive, but the warning was waved off. No one stopped him and no one tried to save his life by preventing him from driving while he was so obviously drunk. He also died in the fiery crash, burned alive in the first few minutes after he wove repeatedly across the center line and crashed at 60 mph into the car carrying Brett.

Some might say that Brett is lucky; he suffered no brain damage. Intellectually he is quite alive—I believe he will go to college one day. But Brett is paralyzed below the level of his second cervical vertebra. His arms and legs will never

move. He cannot breathe at all on his own, nor will he—
ever.

As a specialist in pediatric intensive care medicine, I see
and care for many severely ill and injured children. The
jarring horror of my first moments with Brett ripped a still-
unrepaired hole in the wall of objectivity that usually pro-
tects me from the pain of seeing a seriously injured child.

"He's not breathing," shouted the flight nurse over the
scream of the engine as we unloaded the child from the helicopter and rushed into the emergency department. The
neurosurgeon and I examined the form below us. The cherub
was motionless, save for a grimace when we ventilated him
by mask. "Can you open your eyes?" urged my colleague.
When he did promptly open his eyes we both gasped, staring almost uncomprehendingly at one another, then back to
the figure on the table. The frightened young eyes reached
out so powerfully in their panic that we felt ourselves pulled
to the child. The reality of the nearly unimaginable injury
was upon us.

"Oh, God, it's his C-spine—this kid's a quad." The words
were whispered. They would have been wholly unbearable
if spoken any louder. Even gently whispered, those words
conveyed a sentence of harsh finality known to all in the
room, save one. A few slow, deep breaths and physicians
and nurses resumed control and function: "We're sorry,
Brett. You've been in a car accident. This is the hospital.
We're doctors and nurses—we're going to help you, honey. Don't you have the most handsome blonde hair we've seen
today? This is Tickles, our stuffed bear. Can he snuggle
close by you? He loves little boys." Later Brett and his
father would cry together, as one generation struggled to be
brave for the next, unable to soften the story that had to be
shared.

A portable ventilator now breathes for Brett. The annual
cost of providing his necessary medical and nursing care
exceeds $180,000. The man who caused the accident was
uninsured. The cost in anguish and emotional pain for Brett's

family and for the family of the drunk driver cannot be guessed. The lives of all involved will never be the same.

Although the police report assigned the responsibility for the accident to only one man, we are all to blame. Why do we share this burden? Because we have driven after drinking. Because we have welcomed friends into our homes, entertained them with alcohol, then waved them warmly into the night. Because we have laughed at and accepted public intoxication. Because we have tolerated weak and inconsistent enforcement of drunk driving laws. Because we have accepted lenient sentences for drunk drivers. Because we have conveniently ignored signs of alcoholism in our patients.

Perhaps we can only truly know that which we have experienced. My friendship with Brett has added much to my understanding of the realities of drunk driving and of life. Few intend to hurt or kill others, yet it happens, and the consequences fill our forevers.

I grieve with Brett for the mommy who can no longer kiss and hug away the hurts of childhood, and for the little brother who will not play with him. I share with him the emptiness of a football lying unthrown by the fireplace, of the unopened bag of marbles on the table beside his bed, of the laughing horseplay and the flirtations of young manhood that may never come.

Yet life goes on. I will not demean the resilience of man or child by ascribing to Brett extraordinary bravery or superhuman determination. He is, after all, a little boy. He still laughs and he still cries. He manipulates people and he likes french fries with lots of ketchup. He uses a computer masterfully with a mouth control that also enables him to drive his own wheelchair. Such is our nature, about which Brett has taught me so much: given the slightest toehold, we dig in and we grow and survive. That *is* our nature. Yet with the joy remains the sadness and a certain loss of innocence—even for the physicians who thought they already had the big picture. We survive, but the shocking ease with which beautiful things can be broken haunts us. Twenty-five thousand Americans die each year in auto accidents involving alcohol. Two of them are missed a great deal by my little friend Brett.

# HUMILITY

## Joseph E. Hardison, M.D.

Everybody knows that alcoholics minimize how much and how often they drink. They may deny that they drink at all. Why, even in the face of cirrhosis of the liver, esophageal varices, ascites, and innumerable spider angiomas they may admit to only a "coupla beers" a day. Denial is such a part of alcoholism that it is well known you often have to question the alcoholic's family to get the "true story." Armed with the "true story" and a knowing smile, the persistent physician proclaims, "I told you that guy drinks like a fish!"

A 63-year-old Baptist minister was admitted to the hospital for anorexia and hepatomegaly. He had received the "call" to preach late in life and resisted as long as he could. Finally, he gave up a lucrative position as a company executive and started his own church. It was hard going, but after several years his congregation was loyal and sizable, and he and his family were happy.

He was moderately obese and had adult-onset diabetes mellitus. Ingestion of alcohol was denied. The liver biopsy specimen showed fatty metamorphosis, Mallory bodies, and clusters of polymorphonuclear leukocytes. Diagnosis: consistent with alcoholic hepatitis.

The interrogation began gingerly and progressed. "I want

to ask you again—how much do you drink? Do you drink a pint a day? How many times have you been arrested for drinking and driving? Do you ever get the shakes? Have you ever lost your job because of drinking? Have you ever had the DTs?'' This was answered by calm, flat denial. Wife and daughter, when subjected to similar questioning, answered with hurt expressions, tear-filled eyes, and denials. A slight wavering occurred. The pathologist was questioned again. ''Are you sure this is most compatible with alcoholic hepatitis?'' He was sure. We agreed there was no evidence or history for Wilson's disease, jejunal bypass, or methotrexate ingestion.

The trump card was played for patient and family: ''Your liver biopsy shows strong evidence that you have been drinking . . . that your liver has been damaged by alcohol!'' Denial, frustration, bewilderment, distrust, and anger were manifested by all: physicians, patient, and family.

Then, the pathologist discovered the article ''Nonalcoholic Steato-hepatitis: Mayo Clinic Experiences with a Hitherto Unnamed Disease,'' by Ludwig and coworkers, in which 20 cases of nonalcoholic patients with liver biopsy findings consistent with alcoholic hepatitis were described. Most of the patients were moderately obese, and 25% had adult-onset diabetes. The cause was not found. The authors noted: ''The biopsy evidence sometimes caused clinicians to persevere unduly in their attempts to wrench from the patient an admission of excessive alcohol intake or to obtain a confirmation of such habits from relatives of the patient.''

What a comeuppance! A direct hit to the solar plexus. The sickening feeling of being unmistakably, irrevocably, publicly wrong. The liver reacts to injury in a limited number of ways. We are embarrassed—ashamed. We didn't know. We apologize for doubting—for not believing.

Humility (freedom from pride or arrogance) is an admirable human quality. It doesn't come easily and it doesn't come naturally.

# The Knee

## Constance J. Meyd

We are on attending rounds with the usual group: attending, senior resident, junior residents, and medical students. There are eight of us. Today we will learn how to examine the knee properly. The door is open. The room is ordinary institutional yellow, a stained curtain between the beds. We enter in proper order behind our attending physician. The knee is attached to a woman, perhaps 35 years old, dressed in her own robe and nightgown. The attending physician asks the usual questions as he places his hand on the knee: "This knee bothers you?" All eyes are on the knee; no one meets her eyes as she answers. The maneuvers begin— abduction, adduction, flexion, extension, rotation. She continues to tell her story, furtively pushing her clothing between her legs. Her endeavors are hopeless, for the full range of knee motion must be demonstrated. The door is open. Her embarrassment and helplessness are evident. More maneuvers and a discussion of knee pathology ensue. She asks a question. No one notices. More maneuvers. The door is open. Now the uninvolved knee is examined—abduction, adduction, flexion, extension, rotation. She gives up. The door is open. Now a discussion of surgical technique. Now review the knee examination. We file out through the open door. She pulls the sheet up around her waist. She is irrelevant.

# AN UNEXPECTED BURDEN

## Timothy B. Garner, M.D.

Amid the bustle of my usual afternoon tasks, I had almost
forgotten the earlier call from a physician who was desperate to refer a patient from a distant hospital. I could understand why. The patient had walked into the emergency room
with a severe headache and had quickly developed unilateral
pupillary dilation, had become decorticate and then decerebrate, and was currently barely responsive. A CT scan
showed a large intracerebral hemorrhage needing surgical
treatment. The physician asked for helicopter transport, and
after discussion with our emergency room physicians I requested dispatch of our helicopter and notification of the
patient's arrival.

An hour later, when I realized that I had not yet been
notified, I called the ER.

"John, what's going on with Mr. Jackson?" I asked, my
voice displaying frustration at not having been callled.

"Uh, well . . . your patient is coming by ground ambulance," he said reservedly, almost in a whisper.

"John, I can't imagine a sicker patient than this guy. Have
they been diverted to another call? What is going on?"

"Your guy is coming by ground. I just can't tell you any
more than that right now." John's flat tone and reticence
were so unusual that I decided to talk to him face-to-face.

In the long walk to the emergency room, I cynically decided that this patient was the victim of some political de-

cision—a scenario common in some institutions but one that would have been a first in ours.

I walked into the ER and demanded an explanation. John touched my elbow and said, "Come back here to my office." There, with great difficulty, he said. "We've lost ground contact with our helicopter and smoke has been spotted near the peak of Jonesville Mountain."

I couldn't answer. I found myself looking behind him at the bulletin board bearing pictures of our newly acquired helicopter and its flight crews.

"Teams have been dispatched and a flyover in a few minutes will give us more information."

I was stunned. It was dreamlike, akin to the slow-motion effect just before a motor vehicle accident that many patients had described to me.

"Who's on the flight?" I asked.

A knife stab could not have hurt more when he told me. Two were close friends, and I had worked with the third before she had joined the flight crew.

I turned away, asking John to notify me when Mr. Jackson arrived. During my walk back upstairs, I tried not to acknowledge that Jonesville Mountain is a rugged, often fog-covered peak, the last to be cleared before reaching the referring hospital and Mr. Jackson.

Later, while I was seeing other patients, word came that the flyover had shown a large swath of burned trees and wreckage just below the peak. There appeared to be no survivors.

When Mr. Jackson arrived, I was busy with other patients and a colleague evaluated him, arranging for his emergency operation. He was in extremis but still in much better shape than I had expected—a tribute to the physician who had prepared him for the long ambulance trip. I remained convinced that dispatching the helicopter had been appropriate, but somehow it didn't end there.

By the time the deaths were confirmed and I saw the crash site on the evening news, I was numb. Up to a few hours before, those three had been healthy, caring persons, and now they lay dead, the result of a decision that had been partly mine. All physicians bear the burden of their patients' lives, but this was an unexpected burden. These were not my patients. This burden did not fall into the careful confines of clinical objectivity.

The objectively trained part of my mind adapted new catchphrases to meet this burden: "It was appropriate." "Two other physicians agreed." "The crew knew the danger." "These things happen." Over the next few days, however, my emotional reactions dominated my objectivity. I felt a deep sadness, and inexplicably I felt guilty and responsible. Anorexia, apathy, early-morning wakening, and insomnia set in, despite my best effort to accept what had happened. Soon, even with my limited psychiatric training, I saw the diagnosis clearly, and the burden began to lift; the seemingly uncontrollable symptoms abated. I came away with a much better understanding of situational depression. What helped most, I suppose, was that the mission had been justified.

As I write this over a year later, there is nationwide concern over the safety of hospital-based helicopters. The statistics, like most disaster statistics, do not tell the whole story. Helicopter transport *has* saved lives and lessened morbidity, but the price has been high. I think back to how routine my actions had been that day—how, without a second thought, I had recommended dispatch of our helicopter. How many others act now, or have acted, similarly? How many have cursorily sent requested helicopters, without carefully examining the merits of the trip? And I wonder: can helicopter dispatching, or more important, *should* helicopter dispatching ever become so routine?

Several evenings ago, I left through the emergency room's entrance on my way home—not my usual route. On that crisp fall evening, I found myself in the backwash of our helicopter as it lifted from the nearby pad. Ironically, I realized that one year ago to the day, our tragedy had occurred. I wondered, almost aloud, who will bear the burden, should, God forbid, this one too go amiss? How unexpected and how heavy will that burden be?

# On Deeper Reflection

## Greg A. Sachs, M.D.

Mrs. Smith had been transferred to our geriatrics and chronic disease ward the preceding afternoon while I had been away at clinic. Her lengthy record looked painfully similar to so many others I had read during the first five months of my geriatrics fellowship. She was 87 years old. The chart listed her diagnoses as dementia, pressure sores, incontinence, diabetes, anemia, malnutrition, and multiple fractures. The history did not describe the fractures. Perhaps someone had decided that such detail was not required, given all of Mrs. Smith's other problems.

She was bedridden, responsive only to painful stimuli. A Foley catheter and a gastrostomy feeding tube were in place. Her albumin level was 1.5. She had been in this state for at least three months, as she had been in the transferring hospital for that long after being admitted there in a hypoglycemic coma. The head nurse informed me that Mrs. Smith was hypothermic.

"The temperature is 94.8 rectally," the ward nurse said as I entered Mrs. Smith's room. She cried out, seemingly in pain, as the nurse turned her on her left side. The rest of her vital signs were surprisingly normal, although she was slightly tachypneic. She had many pressure sores, including

large ones on both heels that were still covered by thick,
black eschar.

"My name is Dr. Sachs, Mrs. Smith," I introduced myself. I placed a hopefully reassuring hand on the patient's
shoulder. Her skin was cool and clammy. She cried out as
I touched her. "I'm one of the doctors here on the floor,"
I said. "I'm going to examine you to see what we can do
to help you feel better." I began to examine an open wound
over her right trochanter. I wondered why her previous physicians had bothered to débride this wound while allowing
the sores on her heels to retain their ugly black covering.
The hip sore was two by three centimeters on the surface
but was extensively undermined.

As I moved forward to look deeper into the sore, I thought
I saw movement within the wound. I immediately felt repulsed and feared that there might be maggots in this poor
woman's hip. I saw no organisms, the wound looked clean,
and there was a strange clearness in the center of the crater.
I took a deep breath and looked again at the ulcer. Once
more I noted movement within the sore. This time the
movement paralleled my own motions. I moved closer and
peered deeper into the cavity. Right in the center, in the
deepest portion of the wound, I saw my own reflection staring back at me.

Again I looked to convince myself that I was indeed seeing my own reflection, moving in the wound as I moved
outside of it. I moved the opening in the skin back and forth
to see more of the tissues below. As more was revealed, it
dawned on me that I was seeing myself in Mrs. Smith's hip
prosthesis, the shiny artificial head on her femur mirroring
the image of my face. With her immobility, malnutrition,
anemia, and infection, this sore would never heal. I took
one more look at myself and then left the room.

Seeing oneself in a pressure sore is a stark and frightening vision, disturbing on many levels. In addition to the
grotesque wound and personal reflection, it seemed to mirror the topsy-turvy medical care given to many such patients. Mrs. Smith came from a hospital where she received

mechanical ventilation for a respiratory arrest suffered when she was hypoglycemic. She had pleural effusions tapped and analyzed and innumerable laboratory tests performed. Yet she lay long enough without being turned for all the tissue between her skin and bones to necrotize.

It is sad that somewhere in the course of a dementing process Mrs. Smith lost many of the characteristics that most of us associate with meaningful adult human life. It is sadder still that she received medical treatment that forgot about her as a human being.

It is fitting to have seen myself literally within Mrs. Smith and now to carry a vivid memory of her within me. It is a sharp reminder that I am always inside patients like Mrs. Smith and that they are always inside me; all of us are part of the human community, no matter how demented, contracted, or incontinent. Debilitated and dependent patients need us to reach out and care for them most when we are starting to push them away. It is our distancing of ourselves from these people that is the true dehumanizing act.

Frequently, I have caught myself praying that I would not contract any of the horrible diseases I saw during residency. Now, mostly I pray, "Please, dear Lord, do not let me die with pressure sores."

# UNSUNG HERO

## Lola Oberman

It was a simple operation, quite routine. "Elective surgery," they called it, and there was no reason for apprehension. But things had gone wrong. There had been a nurses' strike, uneasily settled; my x-rays had been lost and had to be repeated; and at the last minute an unexplained change in the OR schedule had moved me up from 10 AM to 8:15.

One does not ask questions. I tied myself into the stiff hospital gown (green for surgery) and bared my flank to the hypodermic the nurse brought in. She checked my gown, undoing the two lower ties.

"Just the *top* tie when you go to surgery," she reproved mildly, and explained, without being asked, "That makes it easier for them, if anything goes wrong. If your heart should stop beating during the operation, they can get your gown off real quick and cut your chest open to get to your heart."

She spoke with cheery enthusiasm, proud of the resourcefulness of the modern surgical team, and I was not alarmed. My operation, after all, was such a simple one. The uneasy feeling in my stomach was probably from the injection or from the realization that my husband wouldn't arrive in time to see me before I went to the OR. No one had told him of the change in schedule.

I became aware of quiet music somewhere, accompanied by a soft shuffle. An elderly orderly, swathed in surgical green with only his ebony face exposed, came pushing a stretcher alongside my bed, maneuvering it with great care, and all the while singing wordlessly in a high, clear tenor a tune that went back to the 1940s. I recognized "To Each His Own" and, already relaxed from the Demerol, hummed along with him.

He had me out into the corridor rolling smoothly along toward the elevator before he spoke. "The Ink Spots," he said. "That was The Ink Spots, wasn't it?"

I thought it was, and we both concentrated on recalling the words while we waited for the elevator. We had it all to ourselves—I couldn't see my companion, stationed behind the stretcher, but we had established a comfortable rapport.

"Duke Ellington," he announced, as if making a statement or delivering a eulogy, and I could imagine him standing, beyond my range of vision, with his hand held over his heart. We were silent in the presence of remembered greatness.

The elevator doors opened, and I was propelled down a long corridor by the best preoperation therapist the hospital could have produced.

" 'In My Solitude,' " he pronounced reverently over my head, and we sang it softly together, humming over the parts we had forgotten, but coming to a strong, sure finish just outside the OR door.

"Your doctor will be along in a few minutes. Then we'll go in."

He disappeared, but I knew he was not far off. I could hear the shuffle of his soft-soled shoes and the almost subliminal music that came from his throat. The tune had changed. Straining my ears and my fading memory, I identified "Harbor Lights." Drowsiness pressed on my eyelids.

"Rosemary Clooney," said the voice at my elbow. I opened my eyes and saw him gazing up at the squares of fluorescent light overhead. "I think Rosemary Clooney did that. Then The Platters picked it up."

He left me again, and I caught a glimpse of the clock as the door to the OR swung open. My husband would be arriving at the hospital just about now. He would find my room empty. Maybe he would meet the cheery nurse who would explain to him about the top tie on the surgical gown.

Suddenly, with the clock face blurring, I felt an urgent need to get a message to him. I must have a trustworthy messenger.

"Hey, Harbor Lights!" I called out, uninhibited enough, in my Demerol haze, to call him by any name that would get his attention, but still conscious enough to be briefly embarrassed by my impropriety.

The kindly face materialized beside me instantly, the head bent to catch my explanation about my husband. Both my brain and my tongue were wrapped in layers of gauze, and it was a struggle to produce the words. I don't remember now what the message was, only that it seemed desperately important at the time, possibly even profound. But it could have been sheer nonsense.

If it was, Harbor Lights gave no sign. He nodded gravely. "I will be pleased to give him the message."

His face floated above me. Then he was gone, replaced by a masked stranger wearing enormous goggles. My turn had come. The door closed, shutting me off from the conscious world. But beyond the door, faint and far off, an ethereal voice was singing: *"Dear Lord above. . . ."*

I knew everything would be all right.

# HOPE BROUGHT HIM HOME

## Ted Kohler, M.D.

Residents tend to be youthful, immature, energetic, impulsive, and idealistic. These qualities occasionally combine to allow them to be more caring physicians than they ever may be again as fully trained doctors. An incident that occurred while my wife, Hope, was a pediatric resident illustrates this point.

She cared for a 5-year-old patient named Billy who had disseminated Burkitt's lymphoma. Appropriate treatments had been tried; all had failed. He lived in Albuquerque, but his mother, an intensive care unit nurse, was from New England. She had brought Billy to Boston to get a final medical opinion, and also to give her family and Billy a chance to say good-bye. While visiting, Billy required hospitalization for sepsis after attempts to keep him comfortable at home receiving antibiotics and pain medication failed. When it appeared that death was imminent, Hope recommended that Billy's father fly to Boston, which he did, assisted by funds raised by family and friends in New Mexico. Billy's condition improved after his father's arrival, despite the fact that his hematocrit was 20 and his platelet and WBC counts were near zero. It appeared that he could survive the trip to Albuquerque. His mother felt strongly that she didn't want to take him home "in a box" and that he should spend the last days with his family in New Mexico. Hope felt guilty for calling the father to Boston because the trip had depleted all the family's remaining funds. She felt responsible for getting them all back home, even though she was somewhat skeptical about the trip.

Billy was too ill to travel without a doctor or nurse, so Hope volunteered to go. The hospital treasurer found funds to pay the plane fare for Billy and his parents. Arrangements were hurriedly made. Hope ran home, changed, picked up a check from the treasurer, and stopped by the hospital pharmacy for a large supply of narcotics because Billy required continuous medication to remain comfortable. Hope left a puzzling message for me at the operating room desk: "Going to New Mexico, back tomorrow."

Because the ticket agent had warned that Billy wouldn't be allowed on the plane if he looked too ill at the gate, Hope wrapped Billy in a blanket to hide his tubes and bloated abdomen. En route to Dallas, he awoke in pain, and Hope administered more Demerol, Phenergan, and Thorazine. Unfortunately, this caused an oculogyric crisis that occurred in the Dallas airport. The gate attendant saw how sick Billy was and refused to allow him to board the flight to Albuquerque. They sent Billy, his parents, and Hope to the nearest hospital, which was a small town outside Dallas. Hope's situation was desperate. She was in the middle of Texas where she knew no one, and she had even forgotten to bring proof that she was a physician. She was responsible for a dying child and two distraught parents who had no money. She began to regret her impulsive decision to take Billy home.

Many of her fears were allayed when she arrived at the hospital, where the personnel were immediately sympathetic. Because they were close to the airport, they had encountered similar situations often. The physician on call gave Hope free rein to do whatever was necessary for Billy, including continuing the doses of narcotics (the hospital's entire supply was depleted by the end of their stay). The nurses were extremely supportive and comforting. They encouraged Hope, telling her she was right to try to get Billy home.

Everyone was deeply touched by the dying child and his parents. One nurse said to Billy's mother, as she rocked her emaciated little boy with his NG tube, "It's just like holding a little piece of heaven, isn't it?" Billy stopped breathing and turned blue. Hope could not hear a heartbeat. When she said, "He's gone," Billy gasped and his heart started beating again. Hope was overwhelmed. She realized that she would have to get Billy to Albuquerque because it seemed he was not going to die until he got there.

Hope spent the next two hours on the telephone trying to get an Army MedEvac, but they could not justify sending a transport for someone whose death was imminent. In desperation she asked if anyone knew a physician with a private plane. Someone remembered Dr. Benson, a young surgeon who had recently learned to fly. Hope called him at 1 AM. After hearing her story, he replied, "Don't go away, I'll be right there." He came with another physician pilot. They spent the next few hours checking on weather, locating a place to fuel the plane in the middle of the night, and finding oxygen tanks that would not explode in the unpressurized cabin. Hope became a little concerned about the size of the aircraft when they asked her how much she weighed. Dr. Benson needed to calculate the time of departure to make sure that they would not reach the mountains outside Albuquerque before sunrise. He had never flown over mountains before. Hope arranged for Billy's parents to leave on a commercial flight that would arrive at about the same time she and Billy would.

The entire evening shift in the emergency room stayed through the night to say good-bye to Billy. Hope boarded the small plane ("like a VW with wings") in the predawn darkness. She held Billy on her lap in the cramped rear seat of the aircraft and struggled to start a new IV before takeoff. As they took off into the star-filled night sky, she had an eerie, surrealistic feeling that she was taking Billy to heaven. Billy awoke briefly, and for the last time, during the four-hour flight. When he asked, "Where am I?" Hope told him, "You're going home now, Billy."

The airport guided the small plane to a spot next to the commercial jet carrying Billy's parents and had an ambulance waiting. As they were preparing to leave for the hospital, Dr. Benson pulled Hope aside and showed her a photograph of his children. "I just wanted to show you why I did this," he said.

At the hospital where Billy's mother worked, the nurses came to Hope's aid. The contents of the NG tube had spilled over her during the flight. The nurses found her a shower, had her clothes washed, and got her something to eat. Billy's family gathered around him for one last time. He died shortly after their arrival.

One month later Hope received a letter from Billy's mother. Enclosed was a photograph of Billy's tombstone, which reads:

Billy D_____
March 28, 1972   Aug 17, 1977
HOPE BROUGHT HIM HOME

# Glossary

AIDS: Acquired immunodeficiency syndrome. A fatal disease caused by transmission of the human immunodeficiency virus by way of contaminated body fluids, most commonly semen or blood or blood products. The virus attacks the body's immune system, leaving it defenseless against infection, from which most victims die.

AGAR GEL: A gelatinous substance actually made from seaweed, used in research and in clinical laboratories.

ALBUMIN: The most abundant protein in the blood, occasionally given as a solution for replacing lost body fluids.

AMINOPHYLLINE: A drug commonly used to dilate constricted airways in the treatment of asthma, bronchitis, and emphysema.

AMNIOCENTESIS: A surgical procedure in which a needle is passed through the abdomen into the uterus to obtain amniotic fluid (the fluid in which a fetus is suspended.) Amniocentesis is often used to detect birth defects.

AMYOTROPHIC LATERAL SCLEROSIS: A progressive, fatal neurological disease in which the patient over several years loses the ability to move, swallow, and breathe.

ANTECUBITAL VEIN: The vein located in the bend of the elbow, where blood is usually drawn.

ANTEGRADE AMNESIA: Partial or total loss of memory due to shock, psychological disturbance, brain injury, or illness. The memory loss is of events that occurred *after* the triggering event.

ANTERIOR TALOFIBULAR LIGAMENT: A ligament over the small front bone of the leg near the ankle.

ARTERIAL LINE: A tiny catheter inserted into an artery to measure blood pressure or to obtain blood oxygen levels.

ASCITES: The abnormal accumulation of serous (from serum) fluid in the abdominal cavity, often seen in liver diseases such as cirrhosis.

ASPIRATION: The inadvertent inhalation of saliva or food.

ATRIAL FIBRILLATION: Uncoordinated rapid twitching of individual muscle fibers in the upper chambers of the heart, causing an irregular heart rate.

ATTENDING: Attending physician.

AUSCULTATE: To listen with a stethoscope for sounds within the body, especially in the lungs, heart, and abdomen.

AXILLA: Armpit.

AXON: The portion of a nerve fiber that conducts impulses away from the nerve cell.

BASILAR RALES: A rattling sound coming from the lower part of the lungs and indicating some abnormal condition.

b-AGONISTS (Beta-agonists): Drugs often used to dilate bronchial tubes in the treatment of asthma.

BASELINE: A known value used to compare values obtained later. Often the baseline is the normal level.

BETADINE: An iodine-containing antiseptic.

BIOPSY: The examination of tissues removed from the body, used to aid in a medical diagnosis.

BLUNT RAKES: Surgical instruments used to grasp tissue.

BOLUS: A large and rapidly given injection or ingestion of medication or fluid.

BRADYCARDIA: An abnormally slow heartbeat.

BRUCELLOSIS: An infection in humans acquired from contact with goats, cattle, pigs, or dogs infected with the bacterium *Brucella*.

BUN: Blood urea nitrogen. A waste product in the blood that is measured to determine kidney function.

BURKITT'S LYMPHOMA: A neoplastic—usually malignant—disorder of the lymphoid tissue.

BURR HOLES: Holes drilled through bone, usually the skull.

CA: Abbreviation for cancer.

CACHEXIA: A general wasting of the body during a long illness.

CARDIAC ARREST: The stoppage of an effective heartbeat.

CBC: Complete blood cell. A measurement (count) of the numbers of cells (e.g., white blood cells, red blood cells) in the blood.

CEREBRAL PERFUSION: Normal flow of blood through the tissues of the brain.

CHEST FILM: An x-ray picture of the chest used to diagnose diseases of the lungs.

CONGESTIVE HEART FAILURE: A syndrome of heart disease characterized by breathlessness and the abnormal accumulation of sodium and water resulting in edema (swelling), which may occur in both the lungs and the general circulation.

CONTRACTURES: A drawing together of, e.g., muscle or scar tissue, resulting in distortion or deformity.

CONTRALATERALLY: Situated on, pertaining to, or affecting the opposite side.

CORD COMPRESSION: The pressing or forcing together of part of the spinal cord, usually resulting in paralysis or sensation loss.

CORTICOSTEROID: A drug used to treat hormonal deficiencies, inflammation, and other disorders.

CPR: Cardiopulmonary resuscitation.

CRANIOTOMY: An operation that involves the cutting or removal of part of the skull.

C-SECTION: Cesarean section. A surgical incision through the abdominal wall and uterus, performed to deliver a baby.

C-SPINE: Cervical spine. The portion of the spine in the neck area.

CT: Computed tomography. A computer-assisted technique for making x-ray pictures.

CYANOTIC: Having a bluish discoloration of the skin as the result of inadequate oxygen in the blood.

CYSTOSCOPY: An examination of the bladder using a viewing instrument inserted into the bladder.

DÉBRIDE: The surgical removal of dead tissue and foreign matter from a wound.

DECEREBRATE: Total loss of brain function.

DECORTICATE: The loss of function of brain cortex where the higher mental functions occur.

DEEP-LINE PLACEMENTS: The insertion of intravenous tubes into large blood vessels deep inside the body.

DEFIBRILLATION: The use of an electric shock to revert an abnormal heartbeat back to normal.

DEMEROL: A synthetic narcotic.

DIABETES MELLITUS: The medical term for the commonly used expression "diabetes." "Mellitus" is pronounced mel'-a-tus, not ma-lite'-us.

DIALYSIS: The process of separating and removing certain harmful elements from the blood, used especially in kidney diseases.

DIGOXIN: A medication often used in the treatment of heart disease.

DILATATION AND CURETTAGE (D&C): The surgical expansion of the uterus and the subsequent removal of growths or other material from the uterine wall.

DIPHTHERITIC MEMBRANE: A patch of cellular debris, bacteria, and deposits that forms in the throat of patients with diphtheria and can obstruct breathing.

DISSEMINATED INTRAVASCULAR COAGULATION: A serious condition in which the body consumes all its clotting factors (often from overwhelming infection) and thus bleeds improperly.

DIURETIC: A drug that increases urine output.

DOA: Dead on arrival.

DOPAMINE DRIP: The drop-by-drop intravenous infusion of the drug dopamine, used in treating shock.

DTS: Delirium tremens. A serious condition of mental confusion characterized by trembling, anxiety, hallucinations, delusions, and incoherence, as the result of alcohol withdrawal.

DTP: Diphtheria, tetanus, and pertussis (whooping cough) immunization.

ECG: Electrocardiogram. The curve traced by a machine (an electrocardiograph) used to diagnose heart disease.

ECHOCARDIOGRAM: The record produced by echocardiography, a technique used to study the position and motion of the heart walls or heart structures by the echo obtained from ultrasonic waves directed through the chest wall. Used to diagnose heart disease.

ECTOPIC BEAT: An irregularly occurring heartbeat out of step with the normal heart rhythm. It is sometimes described as ''palpitations.''

ECZEMATOUS: Affected with eczema-like rash, an inflammation of the skin characterized by redness, itching, and small bumps that weep and later scale.

EDENTULOUS: Without natural teeth.

EDROPHONIUM CHLORIDE: A drug used to diagnose myasthenia gravis; also used in the treatment of myasthenic crisis. See *myasthenia gravis*.

ELECTROPHORESIS: A technique by which proteins can be distinguished by the way they move under the influence of an electric current.

ENDOTRACHEAL TUBE: A soft, flexible tube inserted through the mouth and down the windpipe to aid in breathing.

ENTROPION: The turning inward of an edge of the eyelid.

ER: Emergency room.

ERYTHROBLASTOSIS: A condition indicating the destruction of red blood cells, usually seen in a newborn whose blood type does not match its mother's.

ESCHAR: A dry scab or slough formed on the skin as a result of a burn, a corrosive or caustic substance, or gangrene. Often associated with untreated bed sores.

ESOPHAGEAL VARICES: Abnormally distended veins in the lower part of the esophagus, often a result of cirrhosis of the liver.

ETIOLOGY: The cause of a disease or disorder.

FALSE-POSITIVE: A test result that wrongly suggests that a person has the condition being tested for.

FASCICULATIONS: Small contractions of the muscles, visible through the skin.

FLAME PHOTOMETER: A device used for measuring serum chemistries.

FOLEY CATHETER: A soft, flexible tube inserted into the bladder to aid in the collection or voiding of urine.

FONTANELLE: A soft spot, such as that on an infant's skull, indicating incomplete closure of the skull. A normal condition in young babies.

GASTROSTOMY: A surgical opening from outside the body into the stomach, usually for inserting a feeding tube.

GLIOBLASTOMA MULTIFORME: A rapidly growing malignant tumor of the brain.

GLUTAMINE TRANSFERASE: A liver enzyme.

HEMATOCRIT: The percentage of red blood cells in the whole blood. Useful in diagnosing bleeding disorders or anemia.

HEMIPELVECTOMY: Amputation—along the sacroiliac point—of a lower limb.

HEMOCHROMATOSIS: A disorder of iron metabolism characterized by an excess of iron in body tissues.

HEMOPTYSIS: The coughing up of blood from the lungs or bronchial tubes.

HEPARIN: A drug used to prevent the clotting of blood.

HEPATOMEGALY: Enlargement of the liver.

H INFLUEZAE MENINGITIS: *Hemophilus influenzae* meningitis. A serious infection of the membranes that surround the brain and spinal cord, caused by the bacterium *Hemophilus influenzae* and occurring primarily in infants. It has nothing to do with the virus influenza A.

HISTIOCYTIC LYMPHOMA: A malignant disorder of the lymphoid tissue.

HISTIOCYTOSIS X: A group of diseases of unknown origin, perhaps genetic in origin, characterized by accumulation of abnormal cells.

HODGKIN'S DISEASE: A malignant condition characterized by usually painless, progressive enlargement of the lymph nodes, spleen, and general lymphoid tissue.

HOMEOSTASIS: Stability in the normal body functions.

HOSPICE: An institution for the care of the terminally ill.

HUMERUS: Long bone of the upper arm.

HYPOGLYCEMIA: An abnormally low level of sugar in the blood.

HYPOTHERMIC: Having an abnormally low body temperature.

HYPOVOLEMIA: An abnormally decreased volume of circulating fluid in the body.

IATROGENIC: A disease induced in a patient as a result of a physician's words or actions.

ICU: Intensive care unit.

IN EXTREMIS: At the point of death.

INTERCOSTAL: Between the ribs, the muscles that assist breathing.

INTESTINAL VILLI: The absorptive surface of the intestinal tract.

INTUBATE: To insert a tube into an organ or passage.

ISOENZYME: One of the multiple forms in which an enzyme may exist. The various forms differ chemically, physically, and/or immunologically, but catalyze the same reaction.

IV: Intravenous or intravenously.

JEJUNAL BYPASS: An operation to reduce intestinal absorption—and thus weight—by bypassing the small intestine.

JOULE: A unit of energy.

JVD: Jugular venous distention. An expansion of the jugular vein often seen in heart failure.

LIPOMA: A benign tumor usually composed of fat cells.

LITHOTOMY: A position in which a patient lies on his or her back with upper legs bent perpendicular to the examining table and spread wide.

LITTLE C: One of the subtypes of the Rh blood type, written $Rh_c$.

LOOPS OF HENLE: Part of the microscopic filtering system of the kidney.

LUPUS: Shorthand for systemic lupus erythematosus, a disease of the skin and connective tissue. Often results in severe kidney disease.

LUPUS CEREBRITIS: Inflammation of the brain due to *lupus*.

LYMPHOMA: Any of various abnormally proliferative diseases of lymphoid tissue.

MALIGNANT MELANOMA: A dark-pigmented malignant tumor of the skin that has a strong tendency to spread to one or more sites elsewhere in the body.

MALLORY BODIES: Structures within hepatocytes (liver cells) seen in nutritional cirrhosis (a chronic progressive disease of the liver).

MAYO: A stand on which surgical instruments are kept.

MCBURNEY'S POINT: A point on the abdomen of special tenderness in acute appendicitis. Used as one sign in the diagnosis of the disease.

MECONIUM: A dark green material in the intestine of a full-term fetus that is discharged at birth. An infant born "stained" with this material has probably suffered stress as a fetus.

MEDIASTINAL: The area between the two lungs, containing the heart and great blood vessels.

MENINGITIS: Inflammation of any or all of the membranes around the brain and spinal cord, usually caused by a bacterial infections. See H influenzae *meningitis*.

MERCUHYDRIN: A drug once used in the treatment of edema (swelling) secondary to such conditions as *congestive heart failure* and the *ascites* of liver disease.

METASTASES: The spread of cancer from an original tumor to one or more sites elsewhere in the body. See *malignant melanoma*.

METHOTREXATE: An anticancer drug.

MICROCEPHALY: Abnormal smallness of the head, usually associated with mental retardation.

MYASTHENIA GRAVIS: A disorder of neuromuscular function characterized by fatigue, exhaustion of the muscular system, and often severe weakness and difficulty in breathing, with a tendency to fluctuate in severity.

MYELOGRAM: An x-ray examination of the spinal cord using dye injected through a spinal tap.

MYOCARDIAL INFARCTION: A heart attack. Death of the muscle tissue of the heart, as a result of interrupted blood supply to the area.

NEC: Necrotizing enterocolitis. Inflammation of the bowel, which may result in loss of blood supply to the bowel and may send the body into shock.

NECROTIZE: To cause tissue death.

NG TUBE: Nasogastric tube. A soft plastic or rubber tube inserted through a nostril and into the stomach, for instilling liquid foods or other substances or for withdrawing gastric contents.

OCULOGYRIC CRISIS: A sudden occurrence in which the eyeballs become fixed in one position for minutes or hours.

OR: Operating room.

OSTEOSARCOMA: A malignant tumor of the bone.

OTITIS: Inflammation of the ear.

PADDLES: The flat, metal devices used in applying an electric shock during cardiopulmonary resuscitation.

PANCREATIC ACINI: Microscopic area of glandular tissue in the pancreas.

PECTORALIS MAJOR: The pectoral muscle of the chest.

PEDAL EDEMA: Swelling of the feet.

PHENOTYPIC: Exhibiting a particular genetically determined appearance.

PITTING EDEMA: Swelling so profound that, if pressed, a temporary indentation remains. Often graded from 1+ to 4+.

PLATELET: A tiny disk-shaped structure in blood known chiefly for its role in blood clotting.

PLEURAL EFFUSIONS: Fluid that collects in the space between the lung and its outer lining.

POLYHYDRAMNIOS: An excess of amniotic fluid (the fluid in which a fetus is suspended).

POLYMORPHONUCLEAR LEUKOCYTES: One of several types of white blood cells that help fight infection.

POLYSACCHARIDES: The complex molecular structures found on the outside of living cells.

PRECIPITATES: Substances in a solution that settle down as solid particles.

PRECORDIAL AREA: The region over the heart and lower part of the chest.

PRESSOR TUBES: Intravenous tubes used to deliver drugs to elevate blood pressure.

PRIMIGRAVIDA: A woman who is pregnant for the first time.

PROGNOSIS: A prediction of the probable course and outcome of a disease.

PRURITUS: Itching. Also, the name of various conditions characterized by itching.

PSEUDOMONAL: Pertaining to *Pseudomonas aeruginosa*, bacteria that can cause various human diseases, including pneumonia and *meningitis*.

PVCS: Premature ventricular contractions. Irregular, extra heartbeats that may lead to *cardiac arrest*.

QUAD: Slang for *quadriplegic*, a person having complete paralysis from the neck down.

RALES: A rattling sound coming from the lungs and indicating some abnormal condition. See *basilar rales*.

RENAL SHUTDOWN: Total kidney failure.

RH: A blood type. One may be Rh positive or Rh negative.

RINGER'S LACTATE: A balanced intravenous solution of water and minerals given to mimic body fluid.

ROENTGENOGRAMS: X-ray films.

ROTATOR CUFF: The normal connective tissue surrounding the shoulder joint. Often torn or injured in baseball pitchers.

SEPSIS: The presence of pathogenic—or disease-causing—microorganisms or their toxins in the blood or other body tissue. Usually a severe and life-threatening condition.

SEROLOGIC: Examining the serum for substances, such as antibodies.

SIDEROBLASTIC ANEMIA: An abnormal reduction of red blood cells, characterized by blood cells that contain iron granules.

SIDS: Sudden infant death syndrome.

SOB: Shortness of breath.

SPIDER ANGIOMAS: Little spider-like networks of blood vessels on the shoulders and chest usually seen in persons with long-term liver disease.

SPUTUM: Coughed-up mucus.

STAPHYLOCOCCAL: Pertaining to the bacterium *Staphylococcus*, which commonly causes boils and abscesses and uncommonly causes toxic shock syndrome.

STAT: Immediately.

STATUS EPILEPTICUS: A series of rapidly repeated epileptic convulsions without any periods of consciousness between them.

STEATOHEPATITIS: A condition in which an inflamed liver is noted to be full of microscopic fatty deposits.

SUBARACHNOID SPACE: The space surrounding the spinal cord and brain, filled with spinal fluid.

SUBCLAVIAN CATHETER: A flexible intravenous tube inserted under the collarbone into the subclavian vein and used to withdraw or introduce fluids.

SWAN-GANZ CATHETER: A soft, flexible catheter with a small balloon at the tip inserted into a vein and threaded into the lung's blood vessels. Used for measuring indirectly pressures in the heart. See *subclavian catheter*.

TACHYPNEIC: A state of abnormally rapid breathing.

TB: Tuberculosis.

T-E FISTULA: Tracheoesophageal fistula. An abnormal passage between the trachea and the esophagus.

THROMBOCYTOPENIA: A decrease in the number of blood *platelets*. Often leads to bleeding problems.

THROMBOSED: The formation of a blood clot.

TRANSURETHRAL PROSTATECTOMY: Surgical removal of the prostate or a part of it by means of an instrument passed through the urethra.

TROCHANTER: Any of several bony prominences on the upper part of the femur (between the pelvis and the knee).

UMBILICUS: The navel (belly button).

UNILATERAL PUPILLARY DILATION: The dilation of only one pupil.

VENTRICULAR TACHYCARDIA: An abnormal, rapid heartbeat, which may lead to *cardiac arrest*.

WBC: White blood cell.

WILSON'S DISEASE: A rare progressive disease of the liver due to abnormal copper metabolism characterized by degenerative changes in the brain, involuntary movements, increasing weakness, and emaciation. A pigmented ring at the outer margin of the iris is a sign of the disease.

XIPHOID: The pointed cartilage at the lower end of the breastbone.

# About the Editors

Bruce B. Dan, M.D., is a specialist in internal medicine and infectious diseases. He was the deputy chief of the Centers for Disease Control's Toxic Shock Syndrome Task Force, the American Medical Association's Morris Fishbein Fellow in Medical Journalism, as well as William Benton Fellow in Broadcast Journalism, the only physician to receive that honor. Dr. Dan is now senior contributing editor of *The Journal of the American Medical Association* and medical editor for WLS-TV, the ABC-owned and -operated station in Chicago and can be seen as host of Medical Rounds for American Medical Television on the Discovery Channel.

Roxanne K. Young has been an editor of *The Journal of the American Medical Association* for fourteen years and section editor of its column "A Piece of My Mind" since 1984. She is associate editor of *JAMA* and director of the American Medical Association's Department of the Medical Humanities.